D1092381

THE PHARMACEUTICAL MYTH

THE PHARMACEUTICAL MYTH

Letting Food be Your Medicine is
the Answer for Perfect Health

Gerald Roliz, CNC

The Pharmaceutical Myth is available at special discounts when purchased in bulk for premiums and sales promotions as well as for fund-raising or educational use. Special editions or book excerpts also can be created to specification. For details, contact business@thehealingbody.com

For information or to book an event
contact The Healing Body at
lectures@thehealingbody.com or visit www.thehealingbody.com

Printed in the United States of America

1 3 5 6 9 10 8 6 4 2

Library of Congress Control Number: 2013904654

ISBN-13: 978-1-4819-5440-2 (pbk)
ISBN-10: 1481954407

Book cover concept inspired by Raymond Lee & John Ferguson II
Book cover design by Ulysses Galgo
Interior illustrations created by David Rotman

DISCLAIMER

The concepts and principles herein relate to the promotion and maintenance of health, not the diagnosis or treatment of disease related to physical and/or emotional complaints.

The information in this book is not intended as suggestions for self-diagnosis or self-treatment of mental, emotional, or physical symptoms or ailments. The information contained within provides an overview of the topics discussed, however one should remember that for a complete review of the topic and information discussed, the appropriate texts should be consulted. The notes are intended for use by experienced professional clinicians with a background of education and experience in physiology. Without experience, the notes can be misunderstood, misapplied, and/or abused. The authors take no responsibility for the misapplication of the information in these notes. Results of any product usage may vary.

This book deals with the use of whole food nutrition and herbal medicines to support normal physiology – and certain elements of lifestyle can have a strong influence on physiology.

Any references in the text to specific conditions do not infer treatment for these conditions. The description of any condition within these notes is for description and educational purposes only. The authors are not implying treatments for diseases. Any use of nutritional supplements or herbs is simply given in the context of supplying nutritional and/or herbal support for those with a said condition or without said condition.

No guarantee or assurance of any specific result is given or implied form any suggestions or recommendations herein.

The reader is reminded that regular examinations for the early detection of disease are important.

The publisher and authors are not responsible for factual errors, inaccuracies, or omissions although every effort has been made to use the most current information available. Readers are encouraged to consult other sources.

The statements contained within this book have not been evaluated by the Food and Drug Administration. The products referenced to and recommendations put forth are not intended to diagnose, treat, cure, or prevent any disease. Specific product names have been used to simplify for the clinician the implementation of the principles discussed herein. Any mention of any specific product is the opinion of the authors and not that of the company which said produced said products.

Additionally, the publisher and authors disclaim any adverse reactions or consequences arising out of the use of any of the suggestions, preparations, or procedures discussed in this book.

All matters pertaining to physical and emotional health should be supervised by a duly qualified health care professional.

Practitioners are advised to consult appropriate texts for any contraindications regarding the usage of Standard Process® products and for additional in-depth review of the conditions discussed here within.

There is no guarantee that the website addresses in this book will be valid or correct. Website addresses go stale and sometimes they are taken over by other businesses. There is no guarantee that they will remain valid.

For my mother, who taught me to shine light in places of darkness.

"One of the biggest tragedies of human civilization is the precedence of chemical therapy over nutrition. It's a substitution of artificial therapy over natural, of poisons over food in which we are feeding people poisons trying to correct the reactions of starvation."

— Dr. Royal Lee 1951

TABLE OF CONTENTS

Part II: FOOD AS MEDICINE

Part III: A NEW HOPE

ADDITIONAL

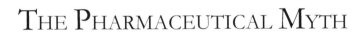

THE PHARMACEUTICAL MYTH

INTRODUCTION

As children, we are given the impression that our medical doctor has the solution to any health issue. This same trust also extends to the government health agencies (FDA, EPA, USDA, AMA) which were founded to protect us, the consumers, from harmful poisons, pharmaceuticals, chemicals and processed foods. Our unquestioned faith has led us to become a fearful nation focused on disease awareness and detection, but oblivious of prevention and resolution. Diseases plague us while health and wellness fail to be restored.

Despite distressing symptoms, lab test after lab test, we are told, "You are fine. All the lab results show that everything is normal." Or we are prescribed a pain killer, yet the medical doctor fails to investigate the cause of the pain. We fill our prescriptions, uncertain if our doctor provided all the information about the possible side effects and risks.

I used to educate medical doctors on the risks of certain medications — side effects, drug-to-drug interactions, liver damage and even death. The doctors were to pass this information to every patient they prescribed a drug for. How is it that I know about medication risks that your doctors have neglected to share with you? I worked as a pharmaceutical sales representative promoting the most popular medications of our time.

In 2001, nearing completion of my undergraduate degree at the University of California, Berkeley, I asked to shadow a former classmate for a day. He spoiled his clients with extravagant dinners, premium seating at sporting and musical events, and weekly golf outings on the company dime. He, himself was provided a fully loaded car, gasoline and car insurance coverage, and a virtually unlimited entertainment budget.

That was the life I wanted, so I worked as a pharmaceutical rep from 2001 to 2006. I promoted commonly prescribed medications, including a proton pump inhibitor (PPI) and a selective serotonin reuptake inhibitor (SSRI), which the pharmaceutical companies referred to as "blockbuster" drugs because of the volume of revenues they generated. I increased the market share of the products I was hired to promote by disguising the risks of medications as safety and tolerability profiles. Because of my exceptional performance, I received quarterly bonuses.

However, after five years, I felt something wasn't right. In every medical doctor's office, I saw sick people sitting in crowded waiting rooms, not getting well. The medical doctors I spoke with rarely mentioned a patient who improved their health. The lack of congruence between volumes of patients taking medications and few becoming well presented me with a large, yellow "Dead End" sign. Time to stop and choose another route in life.

I trained as a Certified Nutritional Consultant and opened my practice. I discovered that many of my nutritional clients had symptoms that resembled the side effects of specific medications. My mission became to increase awareness of specific medications most medical doctors prescribe without full disclosure of their risks. You will gain a perspective on current standards of medical practice in America, as well as how to avoid its shortcomings with wise nutrition.

COMPELLED TO FEAR

While you sit in a medical doctor's office, you are compelled to fear disease because it is what medical doctors are trained to diagnose and what pharmaceutical advertisements subliminally hint for you to self identify.

As a sales rep, I used fear to train medical doctors to recognize opportunities to prescribe the medications I represented. I was trained by my manager to hold out a black and white image of a sad and dejected person with his hand on his forehead and his eyes looking down. I thus alerted doctors to identify and diagnose Major Depressive Disorder for anyone presenting grief or sadness. The suspicion of suicidal thoughts was enough reason to prescribe an anti-depressant. Not just any anti-depressant, *my* anti-depressant.

Fear is the pharmaceutical industry's best friend. For example, the public is currently trained to fear high cholesterol numbers although our bodies produce cholesterol for multiple necessary purposes such as producing testosterone, progesterone and other steroid hormones.

When we are scared, we panic. When we panic, we forget how to rationally evaluate our options. When high cholesterol levels are reported, we must remain calm and ask the next question. Why are cholesterol numbers high? Are testosterone or progesterone levels so low that our body is increasing cholesterol production? Do our bodies really need help converting cholesterol into these hormones rather than cholesterol suppression?

Our fear allows an authoritative professional to prescribe a pharmaceutical to merely change a numerical value without addressing the root cause. Chapter six, *The Illusion of Medicine*, shows how the pharmaceutical industry creates magic with the use of clever advertising. I have written this book to educate you on the cause of illnesses so you may move forward with effective and safe solutions while avoiding the pitfalls of a healthcare system that may prevent you or a loved one from achieving optimal health. Information can turn fear into courage.

OVERLOOKING NUTRITION

We all learned in school that deficiencies in Vitamin C, Vitamin D and iron cause scurvy, rickets and anemia, respectively. [1] In a Nutrition 101 course at U.C. Berkeley, I learned that many diseases are linked to, and possibly caused by, nutritional deficiencies. Even in the news we hear about the connection between Vitamin D deficiency, cancer development and poor bone health. [2,3,4] What if every disease is inherently linked to a deficiency of single or multiple nutrients? Why do medical doctors not assess nutritional health during initial medical exams or annual physicals?

Most medical doctors receive an average of eight hours of nutritional training. Our lack of confidence in their ability to understand which nutrients or foods are lacking from our diet leads many of us to reach for vitamin supplements. We may not know if a particular supplement will work to prevent the onset of a disease, but we have a hunch — a gut feeling inside of us that believes that the nutrients we consume through the foods we eat have some influence on our personal health. Part two, *Food as Medicine* confirms that our gut may have been telling us the truth all along from the very beginning.

HOLISTIC HEALTH CARE PRACTITIONERS

Holistic health care practitioners implement modalities that support your body's natural healing abilities. The body only wants to do one thing when it is injured or ill — to heal.

"Holistic health" describes therapies that treat a patient as a whole person. Practitioners look at an individual's overall physical, mental and emotional well-being in order to recommend treatment. They treat the symptoms of illness by addressing the underlying cause. They also focus on preventing illness and emphasize optimizing health by supporting the natural regenerative processes of the body.

All the body organs and systems are genetically programmed to work well for your entire life. Your body can regenerate and reach a state of optimal health just as easily as it develops ailments or a diagnosable disease. The support of a holistic health care practitioner is invaluable in treating you as a whole person.

I have written *The Pharmaceutical Myth* so you can learn how to converse confidently with your medical doctor about all aspects of your health. Every healthcare professional has developed his or her trade to contribute to the health of humanity. It is my deepest desire for all medical doctors and holistic health care practitioners to increase communication and collaboration with each other for the benefit of their patients' health. I respect and appreciate their altruistic intentions. My goal is to provide you with information to understand the cause of disease as well as tools to restore your health. As we become examples of health and vitality for our children and grandchildren, we give them a better chance to live free of disease and physical suffering.

PART I:

THE PHARMACEUTICAL MYTH

*"All truth passes through three stages. First, it is ridiculed. Second,
it is violently opposed. Third, it is accepted as being self-evident."*

— Arthur Schopenhauer

1

STATE OF THE NATION'S HEALTH

"It is no measure of health to be well adjusted to a profoundly sick society."

— Jiddu Krishnamurti

After school one spring day when I was 13 years old in Clayton, California, I sat on a bench waiting for the public bus. Next to me sat a very small elderly man wearing a nylon jacket and sweat pants. His beanie made him resemble 'Micky' Goldmill, the trainer for Rocky Balboa. His white hair and prominent ocular arches made him look like he was ready to cheer you on as you faced your biggest life challenge.

He turned to me and asked if I enjoyed school. I nodded my head, surprised that I even responded, for I was quite reserved with strangers. Micky noticed that I was willing to listen to him, so he shared how he had lost his engineering job due to a restructuring at his software company. He eventually sold his blue Volvo station wagon because he couldn't afford the monthly payments. He was behind four months in rent. I listened politely, wondering if he was going to ask me for money, or perhaps if he could train me to become America's next great boxing legend.

Instead, he told me that he was diagnosed with hypothyroidism four years ago and fibromyalgia two years ago. His medical doctor suspected he had Type II diabetes. I was completely clueless about these conditions. He told me about meeting with a group of retired men with fibromyalgia every week to read a few poems out of a book. I imagined fibromyalgia was an oddball religious group which studied their own version of a Bible. Or maybe it was a breed of dog and his club was similar to my lunch period chess club.

The bus eventually arrived with no adjacent seats available. Seconds before we boarded the bus, Micky shared one last concern. "My medical doctor thinks he's a god, but I feel terrible. All he does is diagnose me with different diseases and run test after test. But I still don't feel well. Now, he tells me it's all in my head. Why do I even go to the doctor's office?"

I didn't know how to respond. I was rather shell-shocked. My throat swelled like it always did when I had to stand in front of the class and provide a speech. Did he actually want an answer from me, or was he just in need of someone to listen? I tried to respond, but the frog in my throat turned into an inflatable dinosaur, so no word could escape my vocal cords.

As a child, I was taught that if I ever became sick or ill with an infection or had an asthma attack, my mother would bring me to the hospital and the person wearing the white coat would help me feel better. I was trained to believe that a medical doctor is there to address any and all health related issues.

And now Micky, the nice guy who I imagined would train me to box and be ready to stand up to my junior high bullies was making me choke on my words while planting a seed of doubt in the very fabric of my healthcare paradigm. As I boarded the bus, I began to wonder if maybe, just maybe, medical doctors don't always have the ability to help us become well.

Micky's question sent me seeking to prove that going to the doctor's office improved the health of all people. To my surprise, I found the contrary. The United States has a health crisis.

A SICK SOCIETY

Nearly two-thirds of U.S. adults are overweight or obese.[5] The life expectancy of women is dropping each year.[6] In 2011, 25.8 million children and adults in the United States (8.3% of the population) were found to have diabetes and the numbers continue to climb.[7] The American Cancer Society, American Diabetes Association and the American Heart Association report that the human and economic costs from cardiovascular disease, cancer and diabetes is expected to rise.[8]

In 2012, over 1.5 million new cancer cases were expected to be diagnosed and over 577,000 Americans were expected to die of cancer — more than 1,500 people a day. Currently, cancer accounts for nearly 1 of every 4 deaths, the second most common cause of death in the U.S., exceeded only by heart disease.[9]

Despite the development of technologically advanced diagnostic tools and ongoing discovery of "new and improved" pharmaceutical drugs, 785,000 Americans are estimated to have a first time coronary attack each year, while another 470,000 people will have a recurrent attack.[10] Approximately 610,000 people will have a stroke for the first time, and another 185,000 people will have a recurrent stroke as the current medical solutions fail to prevent future cases.[2]

While Micky was a random person at a bus stop, he raised doubts and provoked questions that challenge the current healthcare system. The statistics that measure the growth rates of disease and chronic illness in our society made me realize that Micky was not alone.

There are over 100 doctor offices within a five minute drive from my home. Like many people, there's no need to travel far to reach a medical doctor. They are abundant, accessible and available.

These medical doctors often employ a vast arsenal of pharmaceutical medications and other tools, which they refer to as an "armamentarium." The right to dispense pharmaceutical medications separates the medical doctor from the layperson. The armamentarium represents a deep library, cataloged according to the disorders they are intended to treat. Pharmaceutical companies innovate and regularly add new pharmaceutical medicines to this library, then influence medical doctors into believing these are the key to health and wellness. Unfortunately, the armamentarium is easily recognized as an expanded medicine cabinet with many of its contents containing skull and crossbones warning labels.[*] In fact, over 4,750 drugs are available in the U.S. medical doctor's medicine cabinet in a total of 17,992 drug products, which vary in formulation, dosage and method of administration.[11]

With the abundance of "pharmaceutical options" available to treat a multitude of acute and chronic diseases, why are disease rates continuing to climb for common disorders like diabetes, heart disease and cancer? If we are to assume that pharmaceutical medications are effective in treating today's modern diseases, are medical doctors doing enough to bring disease rates down?

The job of a medical doctor, defined as the 'standard of care,'[†] often requires him or her to provide an ailing patient a prescription for pharmaceutical treatment of a particular disease. American medical doctors prescribe medications at an extraordinary rate. In 2010, Americans were the most medicated people around the globe. Over 61% of the adult population is on a prescription pharmaceutical drug while 25% of all Americans are taking four pharmaceutical drugs or more (see Figure 1).[12] The actual percentage of people ingesting a pharmaceutical is even higher if we account for all individuals who self-medicate with over-the-counter (OTC) pharmaceutical products.

Society has taught us to assume that a prescription given by a medical doctor in times of illness represents the solution for that particular health issue. By extension of this assumption, I set about to

---

[*] The modern day skullcap warning label has now been replaced with "black box" warnings. A black box warning, also known as a "boxed warning" or "black label warning," is named for the black border surrounding the text of the warning that appears on the package insert describing the medication. It is a serious medication warning required by the U.S. Food and Drug Administration (FDA).

[†] Standard of care is a general or specific medical treatment guideline. It specifies appropriate treatment based on scientific evidence medical professionals provide as treatment of a given condition.

Country	% adults taking at least 1 prescription	% adults taking at least 4 prescriptions
Australia	54%	18%
Canada	56%	17%
Denmark	--	--
France	45%	17%
Germany	54%	12%
Netherlands	56%	15%
New Zealand	55%	18%
Norway	54%	14%
Sweden	50%	17%
Switzerland	40%	10%
United Kingdom	52%	13%
United States	61%	25%
Median (countries shown)	*54%*	*17%*

Source: Commonwealth Fund 2010 International Health Policy Survey of Eleven Countries
Source: OECD Health Data 2010 (Oct. 2010)

Figure 1. Percentage of population regularly taking prescription pharmaceuticals in 2010.

find out if the American people represent the healthiest of all populations. After all, since America has the highest percentage of people taking the "miracle" drugs, should I expect anything less?

This assumption was quickly squashed, and the failure of pharmaceutical medicine quickly came to look like an inconvenient truth we don't want to believe.

POOR VALUE IN THE HEALTHCARE SYSTEM

The Organization for Economic Co-operation and Development (OECD) is an international organization that helps governments research the economic, social and government challenges of a globalized economy. In 2007, it found that health expenditures in the United States ranked highest, at $7,482 per person. As a country, we are paying a substantial premium for our healthcare.

If the adage "You get what you pay for" were to apply to healthcare, we should assume that the quality of medical care in the

U.S. is the best in the world. However, the Healthy Life Expectancy of our population falls below 23 other nations.[13] See Figure 2. These numbers are reported by the World Health Organization (WHO), which releases an annual report that figures the number of years that a child born now can expect to live in good health (i.e., total life expectancy minus years of illness to adjust for quality of life).

	Country	Per Person Health Care Expenditure[1]	Healthy Life Expectancy[2]
1	Japan	$2,746	76
2	Switzerland	$4,570	75
3	Australia	$3,351	74
4	Iceland	$3,379	74
5	Italy	$2,769	74
6	Spain	$2,734	74
7	Sweden	$3,431	74
8	Canada	$3,850	73
9	France	$3,667	73
10	Germany	$3,722	73
11	Ireland	$3,533	73
12	Israel	$1,994	73
13	Luxembourg	$4,493	73
14	Netherlands	$4,410	73
15	New Zealand	$2,447	73
16	Norway	$4,884	73
17	Austria	$3,907	72
18	Belgium	$3,423	72
19	Denmark	$3,766	72
20	Finland	$2,909	72
21	Greece	$2,723	72
22	United Kingdom	$3,030	72
23	Korea	$1,645	71
24	United States	$7,482	70
25	Mexico	$836	67

Figure 2. Health Care Expenditure & Healthy Life Expectancy Comparison among 25 OECD nations.

When I first read these statistics, I could not believe the U.S health care system would score so abysmally, especially since our cost is the highest. We spend more than any other country for medical care, pharmaceuticals and other health related services. Although we have the highest percentage of people taking prescription medications, the number of patients diagnosed with chronic disease continues to climb. In the end, our healthy life expectancy is lower than many other industrialized countries. It just doesn't add up. The poor outcome of our current healthcare system sounds like we, the consumers, are either getting ripped off or something is terribly wrong. Perhaps both. One fact is obvious — *we are not getting what we pay for.*

Is the pharmaceutical industry failing us as well as our health? Is there a flaw in the current medical system? Are our doctors hiding the truth by not telling us what we can do to attain vibrant health and wellness? Is there anything we can do differently?

The answer to these and Micky's final question must be uncovered if we as a population are truly to become healthy. More importantly, we must address the cause of any and all physical degeneration. For if we are successful, we can support the natural healing abilities of our bodies and live free of disease. Each one of us has the right to live a healthy life, free of all illness. How do we achieve this?

To begin, we must know the risks and dangers of taking pharmaceuticals and understand why they have failed to improve the health of our population. Furthermore, we must not give up hope and learn how to optimize our health.

I didn't hear no bell.

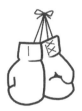

2

ALLOPATHIC MEDICINE

"We need to be confident. We need not to blink."

— Sebastian Coe

On an October morning in 1999, it was so cold that I could see the frost form as I exhaled. I walked across to the east side of U.C. Berkeley's campus for an Organic Chemistry 3A midterm exam. Strolling along College Avenue, I was dreading the 8am meeting with the academic gods who would decide whether I would be allowed into the ranks of medical doctors. Organic chemistry had the ominous reputation of weeding out students who were not cut out for a degree in the life sciences. It was the greatest hurdle to completing the pre-med coursework.

To fail Organic Chemistry 3A, was the harbinger of medical school application death. The pressure to perform well loomed over the underground lecture hall. I found a seat midway down along the left side of the 500 seat auditorium — the chosen seat where I couldn't be distracted by latecomers but conveniently located near the restroom. I sat down, pulled out my pencil and received the test packet from a graduate student instructor who would possibly be responsible for grading my exam. I smiled at her to create a rapport that might later serve to save me academically. Ten minutes into the 90-minute exam, the fire alarm went off, sending a pulsing scream that pierced the eardrums. Everyone had to pack up their exam and proceed out of the building to a safe location.

After evacuating the building, we stood in the morning cold for an hour, waiting for the fire department to inspect the building and give clearance for re-entry. We all herded back into the building to resume the exam with twenty minutes left. I returned to my 'chosen seat,' thinking, "Screw the seat selection theory. I need a countermeasure for fire alarm debacles."

The fire alarm had increased my stress level ten-fold. I assumed that the perpetrator who pulled the false alarm was a classmate ill prepared for the exam and decided to commit academic kamikaze while taking us all down with him.

There is an optimal time and place to use every tool. For a fire alarm, it is not a student "crying wolf" to save themselves from academic probation. It is an efficient use of fire department resources and tax dollars when a fire alarm is used to call for help in response to emergencies, physical trauma or fire, not to cover for being too hung-over from fraternity parties to study.

The application of the right tools at the right time and place also applies to allopathic medicine.

The term "allopathy" was created by a German physician Samuel Hahnemann in the early 19th century by combining *allos* "opposite" and *pathos* "suffering" to represent the use of chemicals to alleviate a patient's symptoms so they no longer manifest a diagnosable disease. Chemical substances intended for medical treatment are referred to as pharmaceuticals, such as laxatives to relieve constipation. Medical doctors who use pharmaceutical medications, radiation and surgery as primary treatment strategies to patient health issues are often referred to as *allopathic medical doctors*. Allopathic medicine is often referred to as *Western medicine*.

Fast acting pharmaceuticals are exceptional tools — an integral part of the life saving process. For example, the EpiPen® supplies a miraculous emergency injection of epinephrine that can save the life of a person in anaphylactic shock due to accidental exposure to food or environmental allergens. My childhood friend, Ricky has had his life saved with the EpiPen® on multiple occasions. He has a severe allergy to peanuts. One peanut would make his face and throat swell, his lungs and airways collapse and his ability to breathe or call for help become impossible. One day, on the school playground, a classmate offered Ricky some M&M's. I saw him fall to the ground and I ran to the school nurse. With the quick administration of the EpiPen®, the swelling abated, his airways opened up and his life was saved. Allopathic medicine's arsenal of fast-acting pharmaceuticals is invaluable for acute and emergency situations.

Allopathic medical intervention has proven to be necessary immediately after acute trauma. If a person suffers a stroke, accident (car, work related) or other emergency, an ambulance can arrive within minutes and escort him to a nearby hospital where heroic medical interventions can save a life from otherwise certain disability or death. One of my uncles had a heart attack a few years ago. The first responders arrived and placed the paddles of a defibrillator against his chest and yelled "Clear!" Just seconds later, his heart was beating again and he was sent to the hospital for rest and monitoring. The ability to restart one of the most complex muscles in the body is an amazing feat, invaluable for acute and emergency situations.

The skills of an experienced surgeon are often irreplaceable in emergency situations. During a childhood birthday party, my older cousin's appendix burst. She began to cry loudly in agony, overlapping her hands and grasping the right side of her abdomen. She was rushed to a local hospital and within an hour she returned home with stitches. The swift removal of her appendix and dangerous toxins that were released averted a very disastrous life situation. For such situations alone, hospitals and surgery are a necessity.

The procedures to cosmetically help burn victims or those with superficial injuries that leave tremendous amounts of scar tissue are another admirable use of modern surgical tools. And implantable devices — pacemakers, hip replacements, prosthetic limbs — have allowed many people to continue a full life. In some cases, the impact of these technological advances improves the quality of life. We hear on the news about the extraordinary examples of young children who undergo leg amputations, then given the use of prosthetic limbs, they develop into the world's most inspiring world class athletes. Medical technologies and the development of allopathic medicine have allowed many individuals to actualize their life's fullest potential.

The ingenious use of technology for imaging and assessment is another great hallmark of allopathic medicine. Modern diagnostic tools depend on technologies that can detect and analyze proteins, hormones and toxins in the blood, urine, saliva and hair. Due to the specificity of such tests, we can even pinpoint which organs require restorative support and to what degree.

MEDICAL DOCTORS AND FIREFIGHTERS

Allopathic medical doctors with surgical skills to close a gaping wound are just as important as firefighters at a six-alarm fire. We can be grateful for their skillful hands if we are involved in a car accident or experience physical trauma. To remove and re-attach various tissues or organs with complete control requires a level of sensitivity and dexterity gained from years of study and practice.

Paramedics and Emergency Medical Technicians (EMT), usually the first medical professionals to reach the scene of an accident, are trained not to hesitate when resuscitating a trauma victim, controlling bleeding and stabilizing spinal injuries. They can administer fast-acting medications as needed. My younger brother works as a paramedic and heroic firefighter to save lives as a public service. In his day-to-day emergencies, he has many success stories applying pharmaceuticals on those who have been delivered a second chance at life.

We should all honor the work of the million firefighters, quarter million paramedics and over 28,000 emergency medicine doctors who apply their skills for victims of acute trauma and life-threatening emergencies with expediency and precision. Unfortunately, some 600,000 physicians spend a majority of their time in direct patient care, employing pharmaceutical therapy at the wrong time for their patients.

The next two chapters will open Pandora's Box of inconvenient truths. Brace yourself. Some may anger you, others will leave you in awe. All will illuminate the risks of pharmaceuticals. Once you understand the risks, you'll begin to realize that maybe your allopathic medical doctor is actually my classmate who pulled the fire alarm when there was no real emergency.

3

Hear No Evil, See No Evil, Speak No Evil... Do No Evil?

"The person who takes medicine must recover twice, once from the disease and once from the medicine."

— William Osler, MD

When I was five years old, I broke out in a fever, sweating profusely to the point of dehydration. My grandmother tucked me into bed and placed a small hand towel soaked in cold water on the top of my forehead. I felt refreshed. When my muscles began to ache, my grandmother was there to comfort me. Even though she spoke only a few soothing words, we both knew that she would support me through this agonizing ordeal. As she sat next to me on my bed, she reassured me that the fever would pass and there was nothing to worry about. Every few hours, she fed me chicken soup she made by boiling a whole chicken for hours. She explained that it contained nutrients, especially Vitamin C and calcium from the bones and cartilage, which would support my body's natural healing processes. My grandmother was the calmest of all my relatives. She, like many grandmothers, knew from years of wisdom that when ill, our bodies always need rest, water and nourishing foods.

She adamantly believed there was no place for drugs. On the day my fever broke, I asked my grandmother, "Grandma, why do people take medicine if they know they will get better after a few days?"

She smiled at my inquisitive nature. "One day, I'll tell you about the discovery and development of modern day medicines. But that day is not today." She never did answer my question. Like any child with an unanswered question, I remained curious enough to research the history of modern medicines and to learn what they are really used for.

The dictionary defines **medicine** as a remedy for the treatment of illness. Conversely, a **poison** is defined as a toxic substance that causes illness, injury or death if taken into the body. These two words appear to be antagonistic by definition. Is it possible for a substance to be both a medicine and a poison?

PANDORA'S MEDICINE BOX

In the early 1900s, livestock in the U.S. were fed a particular type of hay. Some livestock owners found that spoiled sweet clover hay would cause their animals to die of hemorrhaging (uncontrolled internal bleeding). In humans, hemorrhaging may have an early sign as capillaries in the skin breaking down, commonly referred to as bruising. From the effects of spoiled hay, researchers isolated a substance, dicoumarol. Then, in 1948, they patented a synthetic form called warfarin, which sold as a rodenticide (rat poison). Warfarin rapidly became the most widely used rodenticide throughout the world, because it effectively causes rats to hemorrhage to death soon after they ingest it. However, its use as a rat poison today is declining since many rat populations have become resistant to it, necessitating the use of poisons of greater potency.

Pharmaceutical companies now market warfarin as an anticoagulant agent, making it the most widely prescribed oral anticoagulant drug in North America. Unfortunately, the number of drugs reported to interact with warfarin continues to expand.[14]

One person's rat poison is another person's medicine.

Nitrogen mustard was developed as a biological weapon during World War II. The Chemical Weapons Convention (CWC) now outlaws the production, storage and deployment of chemicals in warfare. The CWC identifies substances related to biochemical weapons into three categories:

Schedule 1: Few or no uses other than the use as a chemical weapon.

Schedule 2: Used to manufacture chemical weapons and some commercial products.

Schedule 3: Used to manufacture commercial products and some chemical weapons.

Nitrogen mustard is listed as a Schedule 1 substance. Wounds due to mustard agents resemble burns and blisters, so they are usually classified as "blistering agents". Since they also cause severe damage to the eyes, respiratory system and internal organs, they are also tissue-injuring agents.[15]

Nitrogen mustard is also marketed as Mustargen®, mechlorethamine, mustine and HN2 for cancer chemotherapy. Chemotherapy drugs are "antineoplastic" or "cytotoxic," which means they are toxic to healthy cells. The first patient in the United States was treated with it in December 1942.[16]

One person's biochemical weapon is another person's medicine.

The major goal of the International Agency for Research on Cancer (IARC), part of the World Health Organization (WHO), is to identify causes of cancer. The most widely used system for classifying carcinogens comes from the IARC. Over the past 30 years, IARC has evaluated the cancer-causing potential of more than 900 chemicals, placing them into one of the following groups:

Group 1: Carcinogenic to humans

Group 2A: Probably carcinogenic to humans

Group 2B: Possibly carcinogenic to humans

Group 3: Unclassifiable as to carcinogenicity in humans

Group 4: Probably not carcinogenic to humans

In the IARC database for chemotherapy agents, cyclophosphamide (or Cytoxan®, a common chemotherapy used in multiple cancer types) is classified as a Group 1 carcinogen with ample evidence for carcinogenicity to humans. [17] Most chemotherapies are classified as alkylating agents, which means they are carcinogenic themselves.

One person's cause of cancer is another person's treatment of cancer.

According to classical Greek mythology, Pandora was the first woman on Earth and made out of water and clay. The gods endowed her with many gifts, including a beautiful box she was instructed never to open. However, this taboo fed her curiosity until one day she could no longer contain her desire. When she opened it all the evils in the world escaped to wreak havoc among the people.

As a child, my dear grandmother had sheltered me from the contents of the Pandora Box that was the allopathic medical world. But my curiosity to understand the development of modern day pharmaceutical medicines brought me to an understanding of the origins of certain poisons or what some may consider medicines. What to call them?

I shared my findings with my grandmother and I watched two expressions unfold simultaneously. The first look resembled the struggle a war veteran experiences when he tries to forget the atrocities he witnessed on the battlefield. The second expression was of calm tranquility and unfettered relief. She knew that my research would allow me to clearly understand that if a substance is poisonous, it always remains a poison. Never could it act as a healing remedy. She then cautioned me. "My dear, you have a clear mind and a good heart. You can fill it with more information, but be sure to package it with light and hope, never darkness and despair."

"I promise, Grandma," I affirmed. Although my grandmother passed away while I was young, the lessons she taught my siblings and me were always the same — to be diligent in our studies, learn from our mistakes and, most importantly, always strive to do the right thing.

After she passed, my curiosity to look deeper into Pandora's Box intensified. I found that cancer centers typically have their own pharmacies, which prepare chemotherapy for administration by oncology nurses. As it is extracted from shipping vials and transferred to IV bags for use, there's some leakage into the hospital and surrounding work environments. Prone to evaporation, the airborne carcinogens create an invisible plume that all employees, patients and visitors inhale.[18] Currently, there is no foolproof solution. Oncology centers have separate restrooms specifically designated only for chemotherapy patient use. Nurses and staff are warned to not use these restrooms because excreted chemotherapy contaminates the restroom walls and evaporates into the environment. Of course, the chemotherapy also enters the waste water system of our municipalities.

The pharmacists know the risks of working with chemotherapy, so they outsource the hazardous job of chemo preparation to pharmacy technicians. Female pharmacy technicians must sign a waiver and agree that they are not pregnant, nor will attempt to conceive a child while exposed to chemotherapy agents which are teratogenic, meaning they disturb the development of an embryo or fetus and cause birth defects, including congenital malformations.[19,20]

The highest wages a pharmacy technician can earn are in an oncology pharmacy preparing chemotherapy doses. This increased income is a bit like hazard pay. Perform the dirty work, acknowledge the carcinogenic and teratogenic risks and be remunerated accordingly. Money talks. Unfortunately, it also condones the poisoning of honest and hard working employees.

A few months ago, I ran into a high school friend at a nearby coffee shop. I found out his wife had been working at an oncology hospital as a pharmacy technician for three months. Though she had signed a waiver, I asked if I could share the information I had uncovered. They were shocked and furious. I felt responsible to help them in any way I could. Within two months she had left her job, I helped her find a sales position with an organic nursery that distributed herbs, vegetables, fruits and compost nationwide. She now works outdoors, breathing fresh air and helping her company expand their market. Six months after starting at the nursery, she earned a promotion and also found out she was pregnant.

My grandmother's voice still reminds me to always use information, no matter how disturbing it may be, to help others and bring light and hope into the world.

DOCTORS DON'T WANT CHEMO

In 1986, McGill Cancer Center scientists sent a questionnaire to 118 medical doctors who treated a particular type of lung cancer. More than three-quarters of them recruited patients and carried out trials of toxic drugs. They were asked to imagine that they themselves had cancer. Then they were asked which of the six current trials would they themselves choose to participate in? Of the 79 respondents, 81% of them said they would not consent to take cisplatin, a commonly used chemotherapy drug. Fifty-eight of these doctors found all trials to be unacceptable because of ineffectiveness and the high degree of toxicity to the body.

In the December 1990 issue of the Cancer Chronicles, an article says: "Many oncologists would not take chemotherapy themselves if they had cancer. Even though toxic drugs often do affect a response, a partial or complete shrinkage of the tumor, this reduction does not prolong expected survival. Sometimes, in fact, the cancer returns more aggressively than before, since the chemo fosters the growth of resistant cell lines. Besides, the chemo has severely damaged the body's own defenses, the immune system, kidneys as well as the liver."

It is suspected that many people who "die from cancer" really die from the chemotherapy long before they would have actually died from the cancer itself. A study completed in 1993 by a German bio-statistician found that the overall success rate for most cancers treated with standard allopathic treatment (chemotherapy, radiation and surgery) was just 4%. [21, 22] Thus, 96% of cancer patients treated conventionally died of cancer or from complications related to their treatment. The only type of cancers treated conventionally with higher success rates were certain blood cancers, such as leukemia or Hodgkin's disease, which approached a 35% success rate.

No doubt many individuals have successfully had their cancer go into remission after conventional cancer treatments. Many examples of men and women determined to heal from cancer continue to live life to the fullest. The sheer will to heal as well as the support of positive thoughts, laughter and nurturing relationships all have healing benefits. These intangible characteristics should all be a part of our daily lives, regardless if we have cancer or not. After all, since 90-95% of all cancer cases are due to environment and lifestyle causes, almost anyone can overcome it with proper lifestyle upgrades.[23,24]

Many patients have persevered through the onslaught of chemotherapy, radiation and even surgery to come out on top, at the end of a grueling process. However, we don't hear about the countless family and friends who did not survive the chemotherapy process itself. Personally, I do not have a single friend or family member who was fortunate to survive this form of treatment. In remembrance of Mr. & Mrs. Yen, Sheri T., Lydia C., Bill B., Jane C., Rick T., Auidi O. and all of those who are dear and close to you. May their passing not be in vain.

BETRAYAL OF THE HIPPOCRATIC OATH

Hippocrates, the father of medicine, lived in the early 5th century B.C. The principles of the famous oath bearing his name are held sacred by doctors to this day: treat the sick to the best of one's ability, preserve patient privacy, teach the secrets of medicine to the next generation and so on. "The Oath of Hippocrates" also holds the American Medical Association's Code of Medical Ethics and has remained in Western civilization as an expression of ideal conduct for the physician. See Figure 3.

The classic translation was used for many generations. However, Louis Lasagna modernized it in 1964 excluding these words:

> "I will apply dietetic measures for the benefit of the sick according to my ability and judgment; I will keep them from harm and injustice. I will neither give a deadly drug to anybody if asked for it, nor will I make a suggestion to this effect."

The omission to no longer include food as medicine could be due to a loss in translation. However, it is more likely due to a loss of the healing intention and the growing use of rat poison, nitrogen mustard and other chemicals which allopathic medical doctors refer to as "medicine" or "treatment".

The Hippocratic Oath

I swear by Apollo Physician and Asdepius and Hygieia and Panaceia and all the gods and goddesses, making them my witness, that I will fulfill according to my ability and judgment this oath and this covenant:

To hold him who has taught me this art as equal to my parents and to live my life in partnership with him, and if he is in need of money to give him a share of mine, and to regard his offspring as equal to my brothers in male lineage and to teach them this art – if they desire to learn it – without fee and covenant; to give a share of precepts and oral instruction and all the other learning to my sons and to the sons of him who has instructed me and to pupils who have signed the covenant and have taken an oath according to the medical law, but to no one else.

I will apply dietetic measures for the benefit of the sick according to my ability and judgment; I will keep them from harm and injustice. I will neither give a deadly drug to anybody if asked for it, nor will I make a suggestion to this effect.

Similarly I will not give to a woman an abortive remedy. In purity and holiness I will guard my life and my art. I will not use the knife, not even on sufferers from stone, but will withdraw in favor of such men as are engaged in this work.

Whatever houses I may visit, I will come for the benefit of the sick, remaining free of all intentional injustice, of all mischief and in particular of sexual relations with both female and male persons, be they free or slaves.

What I may see or hear in the course of the treatment or even outside of the treatment in regard to the life of men, which on no account one must spread abroad, I will keep to myself holding such things shameful to be spoken about.

If I fulfill this oath and do not violate it, may it be granted to me to enjoy life and art, being honored with fame among all men for all time to come; if I transgress it and swear falsely, may the opposite of all this be my lot.

Figure 3. The classic translation recited by doctors before 1964.

THE "BENEFITS OUTWEIGH THE RISKS" MANTRA

An old college friend recently graduated and became a licensed ·medical doctor. Right before he began practicing, I asked him, "Why are carcinogenic substances like nitrogen mustard given to cancer patients and non-cancer patients, with diagnoses like Lupus?"

His response was swift and without hesitation, "The benefits outweigh the risks."

I posed the next question, "Why not provide a medicine with ONLY the benefits and NONE of the risks?" An uncomfortable silence followed for a few seconds. His face froze while he searched for such a medicine within his armamentarium. He had spent many years and hundreds of thousands of dollars to study pharmaceutical medications and their effects on the body, but he could not conjure up a single pharmaceutical therapy for the treatment of cancer that had no risks.

I then shared with him the story about my mother. It is a story I had shared only with a few close friends, but on that day, it was an important one for him to hear.

I'm the oldest of three children. My mother was diagnosed with Lupus Erythematosus in 1981, the year my sister was born. She was told Lupus is an autoimmune condition where the immune system produces antibodies that begin to target a person's own tissues and organs. Her allopathic medical doctors told her the cause of her disease was unknown.

For years, she was prescribed prednisone for inflammation. It caused adrenal fatigue, water retention and many other side effects. She lay in bed with pillows below her legs to drain the water back toward her kidneys and then out the body. She was prescribed various pharmaceutical medications to suppress both her symptoms and the side effects of her initial drugs. Eventually her kidneys showed signs of failure and she would one day require dialysis, forcing her to travel to the hospital multiple times each week. Despite the pharmaceutical interventions, her condition progressed. In 1994, she was urged to undergo four rounds of chemotherapy, even though she had no cancer and the cause of her Lupus was unknown.

On the night of March 1, 1995, while I was a junior in high school, she started coughing blood and was admitted into the hospital. The next day, she went into cardiac arrest after drowning in her own blood fluids.

The ER doctors revived her and inadvertently cracked her ribs in the process. They prescribed multiple pharmaceuticals via IV drips and the nurses stabbed her arms with multiple needles, causing her arms to turn black and blue. For the next two weeks she was confined to a hospital bed where a nurse regularly shoved a pipe down her throat to literally suck the (life) blood out of her lungs. Since the ER medical doctors could not stop the bleeding, she eventually drowned a second time.

The *"benefits outweigh the risk"* is the biggest lie an allopathic medical doctor can tell you. It is based upon an arrogant assumption that no safer medicine exists in the world, and perpetuates a myth of excellence.

Instead of reciting the *"benefits outweigh the risks"* mantra, why not admit to patients the truth that you use poisons, biochemical weapons and carcinogenic substances as so-called medicine. Why not steer your patients in the direction where they can find a non-toxic solution to their health issues? Why not point your patients to the direction of a holistic health care practitioner, such as a Doctor of Chiropractic (DC), a Licensed Acupuncturist (LAc), an energy healer, nutritionist, homeopath or bodyworker. Many of them understand the cause of autoimmune disorders and can help.

At her funeral service one week after my mother left the physical world, my friends, family and distant relatives attempted to comfort my siblings and me by extending their deepest condolences. "Your mom is in a better place now. She no longer has to live in pain." I truly believe that where she is certainly must be heavenly and abundant in all its unimaginable wonders. I accept and appreciate those kind reminders. However, I find it extremely difficult to accept the words, *"she no longer has to live in pain."* Why does any person have to live in pain while they live out their human experience? Why do we condone such suffering? Why do we condone the use of poisons as medicines, especially when the risks clearly outweighed the benefits in her situation?

Nobody *has* to live in pain.

Nobody *has* to die in order to be free of pain.

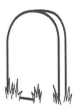

4

THE THREE MAJOR RISKS

"Every drug increases and complicates the patient's condition."

— Robert Henderson, M.D.

When my wife and I are picking a movie to watch, there's always a long drawn out process to identify which one will satisfy us that particular evening. It's an arduous assessment of risks for spending two hours that could make us feel really good or force us down a road of disappointment.

"What movie do you want to watch?" she asks.

"Anything is fine with me, Honey. Have your friends recommended anything? Have you looked at the movie ratings?" I gracefully hand the decision over to her.

"Those ratings are never accurate. They only lead to disappointing outcomes. Remember that Korean movie we saw? We thought it would be a love story, but at the end everyone suddenly died. So depressing."

"But Korean dramas almost always end with someone dying," I said, realizing that everyone dies in real life as well — maybe just not as quickly as they do in Korean flicks.

"Yeah, but why would you want to watch a movie if you know you were going to be left with emotional pain? Remember the last movie you picked? It made me throw up." Apparently, she still hadn't forgiven me for the airplane documentary that gave her motion sickness.

"Alright, how about a horror movie?"

"No. I don't want to have difficulty falling asleep." Insomnia was a side effect of horror films.

I took a shot, "How about Iron Man 2. I heard the special effects are pretty good." It was a risky move, but I've loved comic book characters ever since I was a kid.

"No. Nothing with the word 'Man' in it. You Americans love movies with 'Man'. Batman, Superman, Spiderman, Iron Man. In China, nobody cares about these phony boloney superpowers. It's like you and your people have this false hope that one day the world would be better if you woke up and discovered you possessed some magic power." My wife brought our cultural differences into the decision making. In China, not many kids have heard of Marvel superheroes. I wasn't going to press any further.

Then she decided, "Let's watch 'Love and Other Drugs'. I heard it depicts how pharmaceutical sales representatives sell drugs to medical doctors pretty well."

I was in awe, "So you don't want to watch a movie that will make you throw up, cause insomnia, over-embellish a hero's magical powers and lead to a disappointing outcome. But you want to watch a movie about the pharmaceutical industry. Interesting..."

"Well, it stars Anne Hathaway. I'm addicted to her. She's gorgeous. Help me find the movie." She turned around and went to look for it before I could ask about her addiction to movie stars.

Speaking of which, addiction is one of the three major risks of taking any pharmaceutical. The other two are the unintended side effects and liver damage or kidney failure. Like a poorly produced movie, none of these risks are any fun and they occur more often than we expect.

RISK 1: WITHDRAWAL SYNDROME (AKA ADDICTION)

As you continue to read this section, DO NOT STOP ANY medication without the guidance of the prescribing medical doctor. Our bodies have the potential to become addicted to certain pharmaceutical medications. Patients who stop the usage often report symptoms that are associated with withdrawal syndrome. Always consult your prescribing physician for dosage adjustments of your medications. The effects of suddenly stopping a medication can be fairly dangerous.

Amy, a client of my clinic, was 36 years old when she came in for her first nutritional evaluation. She was recently married and planned on becoming pregnant. She wanted to improve her fertility. During the initial assessment, I saw she was prescribed an anti-depressant and had recently started a new blood pressure lowering medication.

By working together to make lifestyle and nutritional upgrades, we were able to lower her blood pressure naturally. To prevent her from developing low blood pressure, I instructed her to see her physician to have her dosages altered.

Unfortunately, she decided to stop her blood pressure medication on her own cold turkey, without the help of her prescribing physician. The following day, she experienced extreme dizziness, lightheadedness and increased heart rate. She immediately contacted her medical doctor for an emergency appointment. She explained, "As soon as I stopped the medication I became dizzy and lightheaded." Her medical doctor informed her that those were symptoms from withdrawal.

A **withdrawal syndrome**, also called discontinuation syndrome, occurs when a person suddenly stops taking or reduces the dosage of some types of medications after the body has become addicted to it.

The risk for addiction increases with dosage and length of use for each particular pharmaceutical agent.

The body's defense mechanism against poisoning is to develop drug tolerance over time, which leads it to physical dependence. Withdrawal symptoms are often crippling, as the body becomes unable to operate without the substance.

Here is a partial list of withdrawal symptoms:

* Sweating
* Racing heart
* Palpitations
* Muscle tension
* Tightness in the chest
* Difficulty breathing
* Tremor
* Nausea, vomiting, or diarrhea
* Infantile feelings: temper tantrums, intense needs, feelings of dependency, and a state of near paralysis.
* Insomnia
* Mental confusion

* Vagueness
* Irritability
* Anxiety
* Depression
* Tingling in hands and feet
* Intestinal disorders, cramps
* Headache
* Seizure
* Heart attack
* Stroke
* Hallucinations
* Delirium tremens (DTs)
* Cold symptoms (sore throats, coughing as the lungs begin to clear, respiratory problems)

To complicate matters, Amy was taking Paxil® a common anti-depressant medication, known generically as paroxetine, which has the highest rates of all pharmaceuticals to cause withdrawal syndrome.[25] More reports have been filed on this pharmaceutical than any other drug.

With an additional three months of nutritional work, Amy's depression and anxiety improved. She then asked me, "Is it possible to come off this medication? I've been trying for years now."

I explained that the potential for withdrawal syndrome is much greater when psychotropic drug dependence develops, so her prescribing physician is the preferred person to guide her off the medication. The body's neurotransmitter receptor sites develop a physiological expectation of the chemical to be present. If a person misses a dose or suddenly discontinues drug use, these receptors "go hungry" and begin firing erratically which leads to the symptoms of withdrawal.

Many of the other anti-depressant drugs, both selective serotonin reuptake inhibitors (SSRI) and serotonin norepinephrine reuptake inhibitors (SNRI) are reported to cause a high level of physical dependence. Effexor® (venlafaxine) is the second most addictive in terms of withdrawal syndrome.[26]

Figure 4 lists commonly prescribed medications known to cause withdrawal syndrome. This is a partial list, so be sure to consult with your medical doctor on the addictive nature of the medications you are prescribed.

Sadly, women who take pharmaceuticals while pregnant expose their fetus to these chemicals. While in utero, the fetus is fed via the placenta with drugs from the mother's bloodstream. The newborn baby, no longer receiving the drug, may present symptoms of withdrawal.[27] Pregnant mothers or soon to be pregnant women should always speak with their medical doctor about the risk of withdrawal syndrome for the mother and the child. Since Amy wanted to conceive, working with her medical doctor to come off the Paxil® became a priority for the sake of her future baby. When she approached her prescribing physician, she discovered that he had very little experience in helping patients come off addictive medications. I referred her to a medical doctor I collaborate with, and within six months she was finally healthy and drug free. Three months later, Amy became pregnant and was glad that her baby would not have to face the risk of experiencing withdrawal after birth.

Reminder: Do NOT discontinue any medication without the support of the prescribing medical doctor. While some medications may be titrated (progressively adjusted) downward in a few days with no problems, others have been known to require months.

Antidepressants:
- SSRIs: Paroxetine (Paxil®), Sertraline (Zoloft®), Fluoxetine (Prozac®), Citalopram (Celexa®), Escitalopram (Lexapro®)
- SNRIs: Venlafaxine (Effexor®), Buproprion (Wellbutrin®), Duloxetine (Cymbalta®)
- MAOIs: Isocarboxazid (Marplan®), Phenelzine (Nardil®), Tranylcypromine (Parnate®)

Anti-anxiety:
- Benzodiazepines: Diazepam (Valium®), Lorazepam (Ativan®), and Alprazolam (Xanax®)
- Zopiclone and Zolpidem

Blood Pressure Medications:
- Beta Blockers: Atenolol, Propranolol, Acebutolol, Metoprolol, Alprenolol, Bucindolol, Carteolol, Carvedilol, Labetalol, Nadolol, Oxprenolol,
- Penbutolol, Pindolol, Sotalol, Timolol, Eucommia bark (herb), Betaxolol, Bisoprolol, Celiprolol, Esmolol, Nebivolol
- Alpha-Adrenergic Agonists: Clonidine, Guanfacine, Guanabenz, Guanoxabenz, Guanethidine, Xylazine, Tizanidine, Methyldopa, Fadolmidine

GABA Agonists:
- Isoproterenol, Buspirone (BuSpar®), Aripiprazole (Abilify®), Buprenorphine, Norclozapine
- Gabapentin (Neurontin®)

Antipsychotics:
- Clozapine (Clozaril®), Risperidone (Risperdal®), Olanzapine (Zyprexa®), Haloperidol (Haldol®)

Glucocorticoids:
- Hydrocortisone (cortisol), Cortisone acetate, Prednisone, Prednisolone, Methylprednisolone, Dexamethasone, Betamethasone,
- Triamcinolone, Beclometasone, Fludrocortisone acetate, Deoxycorticosterone acetate (DOCA), Aldosterone

Antiepileptic's:
- Valproate (Depakote®), Lamotrigine (Lamictal®), Tiagabine (Gabitril®), Vigabatrin (Sabril®), Oxcarbazepine (Trileptal®), Topiramate (Topamax®), Carbamazepine

Hormone Replacement Therapy
- Estrogen, Progesterone

Figure 4. Partial list of pharmaceuticals known to cause withdrawal syndrome.

> **Food for Thought:** Did you know the word 'doctor' is derived from the Latin, *docēre*, which literally means "to teach." Your medical doctor is more than happy to live up to the deeper meaning of the title and is willing to teach you about the pharmaceutical medications he or she prescribes you. The only challenge is: they are waiting for you to ask.

<u>Question #1 to ask your allopathic medical doctor:</u>
Are the specific pharmaceutical medications you are prescribing addictive?[‡]

<u>Question #2 to ask your allopathic medical doctor:</u>
Do you have any experience helping patients come off addictive pharmaceuticals?

RISK 2: ADVERSE REACTIONS (AKA SIDE EFFECTS)

At the grocery store, an elderly woman named Margaret mentioned that during her most recent doctor's office visit her medical doctor refilled prescriptions for fourteen different medications. She believed that a few of her drugs made her side effects worse. She told her medical doctor, so he switched her to a different set of drugs. Now she can no longer tell which of the new drugs causes which of her side effects.

Each side effect represents an unexpected change in the body that was never intended to occur. ALL drugs have side effects. Unfortunately, they occur more often than we realize. In the U.S., only 1% of drug side effects are reported to the FDA.[28] Hospital consultants report only 1 in 20 drug adverse reactions.[29] Many "known" side effects from taking pharmaceuticals exist, but a greater

---

[‡] At the end of this book is a complete list of all the important questions your doctor will gladly answer for you.

number of "unknown" reactions can occur.

Hearing of her side effects, Margaret's medical doctor is responsible for reporting them to the FDA's Adverse Event Reporting System (AERS). Between its inception in 1969 and 2002, the AERS received approximately 2.3 million reports of side effects on more than 6,000 pharmaceutical drug products.[30] In 2006, the FDA Center for Drug Evaluation and Research recorded 471,000 safety reports via AERS and issued 16 public health advisories (descriptions of safety concern with recommended actions).[31] Public health advisories are warnings directly addressed to the public about the precautions to take when using specific pharmaceuticals.

Most adverse events, however, are not reported and about 10% of patients will suffer harm caused by avoidable side effects.[32] If a person takes multiple medications, they are at increased risk for harm by any one of them because potential drug-to-drug interactions increase. Poor Margaret explained to me how her medical doctor coaxed her into continuing to take all fourteen medications. The methods she explained to me follow exactly how most medical doctors have been trained.

They typically do one of the following:

1. **Immediately lower the dose,** then titrate upward over time to the target dose. This allows the patient's body to adjust to the chemical so that the side effects are not as abrupt (yet may still be present).

2. **Assure the patient that the side effect will disappear over time**. Typically, the time frame given is two weeks. Unfortunately, many patients will learn to accept and live with the side effect.

3. **Add an additional drug to treat the side effect**. The pharmaceutical companies prefer this strategy, because it leads to higher sales and greater profits. Not surprisingly, it is nearly impossible to predict whether a new side effect will result from taking a second pharmaceutical medication.

Once a patient begins to take the second pharmaceutical, more interactions leading to other unwanted side effects can develop. Your medical doctor will gladly prescribe additional pharmaceutical medications. I gave Margaret my card and I let her know that when she is ready to try something different, she can contact me.

SIDE EFFECTS DEVELOP OVER TIME

If a frog is placed in boiling water, it will immediately jump out. But if it is placed in cold water that is slowly heated, it will not perceive the danger and will be cooked to death. Likewise, we may be aware of side effects that develop immediately after starting a prescription drug. However, many side effects take months or years to develop. By then, the side effect may be so severe, it could be difficult to undo.

Joanne was a mother of three when she was diagnosed with osteoporosis in 1999 by her medical doctor. She was immediately prescribed Fosamax® to improve her bone density scans. After taking the medication for seven years, she went for a walk at the park near her home along a trail covered lightly with gravel. After fifteen minutes, as she took a step, her femur (the longest bone in the leg connecting the hip to the knee) snapped in half. "CRACK!" The snap was loud and forever imprinted in Joanne's mind. The pain was excruciating as she lay on the ground waiting for the ambulance. The paramedics hiked in and transported her to the hospital where surgeons immobilized the leg with metal rods and nails. She was bedridden and in pain for six months. Joanne later found out that her medications caused her bone to become more brittle with every pill she took, increasing its chance of snapping.

It is a mistake to assume that all side effects occur immediately after starting a pharmaceutical drug. Side effects may develop over years, even after following the medical doctor's orders exactly. The bisphosphonate drugs (such as Boniva®, Fosamax®, Actonel®) are prescribed to patients diagnosed with osteoporosis. Researchers have found that these bone drugs trigger the body to deposit more minerals into the bone, but do not repair its micro-architecture, which is primarily strengthened by a specific protein, Type 1 Collagen.

Seventy percent of the strength of a bone is dependent upon the quality and layout of the protein-based micro-architecture.

According to reported side effects, patients who have taken a bisphosphonate drug for five or more years may randomly experience a complete fracture of the femur while engaging in normal daily movements. [33] In a healthy person, the femur is the thickest and strongest bone in the body. It also is the bone that has the most amount of bone marrow, which produces white blood cells for your immune system.

With bisphosphonate drugs, the osteoclasts (cells that help break down old bone cells) are poisoned. This allows osteoblasts (which build bone) to stuff the bone with more minerals. However, as a bone becomes denser with minerals, the protein micro-architecture is not renewed, and the bone loses flexibility. This allows it to snap with minimal stress.

Another side effect of bisphosphonate drugs is osteonecrosis (rotting away) of the jaw. This can occur after just two years on the drug. [34]

Most medical doctors are aware of these risks, yet continue to ignore the biological processes that restore the protein micro-architecture of bone. Because of the known risks for rotting of the jaw and femur fractures, they recommend a patient remains on a bisphosphonate drug for no more than five years. However, after five years, few patients, if any, have had their osteoporosis completely cured.

After Joanne recovered from her femur fracture, she came into my clinic. We upgraded her lifestyle and nutrition to address the causes of her osteoporosis, one of which was long-term use prednisone. Prednisone is a synthetic version of cortisol and known to cause osteoporosis. [35] When it is too high in the blood stream, it begins to break down protein in the bone as part of its catabolic (breaking down of tissue) mechanism. Prednisone may have gradually broken down the protein in bone, skin and other connective tissue throughout Joanne's body, given her prolonged use.

It is very important to be aware of ALL the possible side effects of every pharmaceutical medication you are taking.

Joanne had her medical doctor wean her off medications while she and I optimized her diet with nutritious whole foods to support her spleen, liver and endocrine glands which all are important for building strong bones. She drank more water, increased her protein intake and engaged in weight bearing exercise. Over a period of two years, she reversed her osteoporosis and no longer fears running in the park or lifting heavy objects. She has never had to take another medication. But if she did, she would definitely ask her medical doctor to present her with all immediate and long-term known possible side effects.

Question #3 to ask your allopathic medical doctor:
What are the known side effects for each of the prescribed medications?

Food for Thought: You can research the known side effects of any pharmaceutical medications on your own from the following sources:

1) **ePocrates** (www.epocrates.com). This is an online resource where you can access the known 'adverse reactions' and all other information about any pharmaceutical drug, including the risks and potential side effects. ePocrates is also available as a smartphone application, which is very easy to navigate. Information on ePocrates is constantly updated and it is the preferred choice for the most up-to-date information.

2) **Package Insert**. This is the tiny folded white piece of paper that accompanies every filled prescription. Unfortunately, the font is so small that you may need a magnifying glass to read it. Alternatively, the package insert is almost always available online at the drug manufacturer's website as a PDF file.

3) **Purchase a Physician Desk Reference.** Unfortunately, the information is only updated annually and this large book requires a lot of shelf space.

THE SIDE EFFECT MERRY-GO-ROUND

I attended a picnic during the summer of 2012 and watched the twin daughters of my friend, who is a Doctor of Chiropractic, play in the park. Both of the girls, nearly equal in height and weight, were climbing on the merry-go-round. They ran around it on opposite sides, pulling the metal bars. They ran as fast as they could, kicking up a cyclone of dust and increasing the centripetal acceleration of the spinning metal platform. As soon as they reached their maximum velocity, they pulled themselves onto the platform with the strength of their arms and hung on for dear life while screaming in joy. Then, their father came by and spun the merry-go-round even faster. They shouted, "Faster! Faster!" Until their arms gave way and they both flew onto the sand. They stood up quickly and wanted another spin.

After my friend finished another round, I saw the back of his t-shirt, which read:

> *"I take Aspirin for the headache caused by the Zyrtec® I take for the hay fever I got from Relenza® for the uneasy stomach from the Ritalin® I take for the short attention span caused by the Scopolamine I take for the motion sickness I got from the Lomotil® I take for the diarrhea caused by the Xenical® for the uncontrolled weight gain from the Paxil® I take for the anxiety from Zocor® I take for my high cholesterol because exercise, a nutritious diet, regular acupuncture and chiropractic care are just too much trouble."*

This statement highlights the irony of assuming one pharmaceutical medication, like Dr. Erhlich's fictional magic bullet, possesses the universal capability of solving all our health problems. Since all pharmaceutical drugs are known to produce side effects, the magic bullet panacea can never pan out. Even though prescription pharmaceuticals may not be as joyous as riding a merry-go-round, allopathic medical doctors do not mind pushing the physical limits of the human body by increasing the number of prescribed pharmaceuticals. We must always be cautious because eventually something is going to give out.

RISK 3: LIVER & KIDNEY DAMAGE

Joe is a 58-year-old gentleman who came to my clinic in 2010. He was diagnosed by his medical doctor with Gynecomastia, the abnormal development of large mammary glands in males resulting in breast enlargement. Colloquially, this condition is known as "man boobs."

Joe told me, "I never had man boobs. Now everywhere I go, I have to wear a jacket to cover them up. It's bad enough to hang out with the guys and get laughed at. But my medical doctor doesn't know the cause. He said that there is the option of surgery to remove the lymph tissue in my chest." Joe did not want to go in for surgery, which is why he came in for a nutritional evaluation.

During Joe's initial nutritional evaluation, I found the culprits among his pharmaceutical medication history. His medication cocktail included:

- Aspirin®
- Maxzide®
- Diltiazem
- Nexium®
- Ipratropium
- Astelin®
- Malarone®
- Zetia®

- Cipro®
- Zithromax®
- Rapaflo®
- Viagra®
- Levoxyl®
- Ambien®
- Lipitor®
- Flonase®

By searching the clinical archives in the US National Library of Medicine at the National Institutes of Health (www.pubmed.gov), I found Gynecomastia was a side effect of Diltiazem and a few of his other drugs.[36,37] "How is that possible?" He asked.

The metabolism and excretion of pharmaceutical medications primarily involves the liver and kidneys, the two organs most responsible for breaking down pharmaceuticals and other chemical toxins, so they can be removed from the body. The kidneys will take on more of the detoxification load if the liver becomes fatigued, and the liver will help out the kidneys if they become stressed. When both of these organs are fatigued, damaged or clogged, pharmaceuticals and other toxins are diverted to other tissues for detoxification, including the lymph tissue, lungs and skin.

Joe's lymph tissue was serving as the backup organ of detoxification and it too, was clogged, presenting as swollen mammary glands. "Joe, many of your medications are known to inhibit the liver's ability to detoxify various pharmaceuticals, forcing the kidneys and lymph to compensate. In your situation, they are getting stuck in the lymph tissue in your breasts. It's not to worry. We can clear them out of there without surgery."

I noticed Joe's scented deodorant or anti-perspirant, so I asked if he had body odor.

"Yes. I've had it ever since I started taking these medications. This is why I apply anti-perspirant every morning. Is it related?"

Unpleasant body odor is indicative of the body removing toxins via the lymph tissue. Lymph nodes under the armpit remove toxins to the outside world. Anti-perspirants and most deodorants prevent the lymph from releasing these toxins. This forces the body to retain them, which may lead to more severe health issues down the road, including swollen lymph nodes in other parts of the body.

I suggested that Joe speak with his medical doctor to ask if he could decrease the dosages of the drugs creating the most stress on his liver and kidneys. Then we could begin to support those detoxification organs.

Most pharmaceutical medications are excreted by the Cytochrome P450 (CYP450) enzyme system, which includes many different enzymes. Many medications, however, inhibit these enzymes and prevent the liver from removing chemicals.

Joe and I worked with his prescribing doctor to lower the doses of specific pharmaceutical medications. He made nutritional upgrades to support his detoxification organs, including the liver, kidneys and lymph system, draining chemical toxins that were clogging his organs. Within three months, his under arm odor was completely gone and his breast tissue had normalized, so he could wear skin-tight clothing in public again.

It is important to know how much stress each pharmaceutical medication creates on the liver and kidneys.

<u>Question #4 to ask your allopathic medical doctor</u>:
**Do any of the prescribed medications inhibit my liver and
kidney's ability to excrete toxins or increase the level of physical
stress on my detoxification organs?**

Food for Thought: You can research whether your liver or
kidneys are being stressed by any pharmaceutical medications
on your own:

Log into ePocrates (www.epocrates.com).

Search for the pharmaceutical drug, then click the
"pharmacology" tab on the drug monograph. Find the section
that discusses the "excretion" pathways of the medication. The
excretion pathways indicate what percentage of the drug is
eliminated through the bile and what percentage is removed via
the urine. If a drug is primarily eliminated through the bile, it is
creating additional stress on the liver. If the medication is
excreted via the urine, the kidneys are under additional stress.

DRUGS ARE #1 CAUSE OF LIVER FAILURE

Acetaminophen is the #1 cause of acute liver failure cases in the
U.S.[38,39] Acetaminophen is the active ingredient in Tylenol®, which is
available over-the-counter, and one of the most frequently prescribed
medications by allopathic medical doctors (see Figure 5).[40] It is
possible for patients to die suddenly, with no warning, from acute
liver failure (known specifically as fulminant liver failure).[41,42,43]

Though the FDA was established to protect consumers from
harmful substances in our food and drug supply, they allow retail
pharmacies to sell this drug despite its known risks of causing extreme
liver damage. Who is accountable for this toxic debacle? Should we
point fingers at the pharmaceutical companies who manufacture and

	Dispensed Medication	Rx (in millions)
1	hydrocodone/**acetaminophen**	**131.2**
2	simvastatin	94.1
3	lisinopril	87.4
4	levothyroixine sodium	70.5
5	amlodipine besylate	57.2
6	omeprazole (RX)	53.4
7	azithromycin	52.6
8	amoxicillin	52.3
9	metformin HCL	48.3
10	hydrochlorothiazide	47.8
11	alprazolam	46.3
12	Lipitor®	45.3
13	furosemide	43.4
14	metoprolol tartrate	38.9
15	zolpidem tartrate	38.0
16	atenolol	36.3
17	sertraline HCL	35.7
18	metoprolol succinate	33.0
19	citalopram HBR	32.1
20	warfarin sodium	32.0
21	oxycodone/**acetaminophen**	**31.9**
22	ibuprofen (RX)	31.1
23	Plavix®	29.5
24	gabapentin	29.3
25	Singulair®	28.7

Source: IMS Health, National Prescription Audit, Dec 2010

Figure 5. Top Medications by Prescription in the US for the year 2010.

market acetaminophen? Do we blame the drug dealers (medical doctors and pharmacists)? Or do we point fingers at the FDA whose primary responsibility is to protect the American consumer?

Why is acetaminophen still legal to prescribe? Maybe not enough people have died from it. In my neighborhood there is a 4-way intersection with no stop sign. Drivers race through it so fast that crossing the street is unsafe. Though the need for a stop sign is obvious, city officials will only install a stop sign after someone has been killed or run over. This same disregard for protecting the public applies to acetaminophen. How many people will have to die before the FDA issues a court order to withdraw it?

Not all pharmaceuticals lead to liver failure and death. But inevitably most of them will clog or fatigue the detoxification organs, causing discomfort or abnormal physical symptoms.

"WE NEED TO BE MORE AGGRESSIVE"

When the first pharmaceutical does not restore normal and healthy function to the body, a medical doctor will often prescribe an additional one. This indicates that the first drug prescribed did not work. But the patient is told, "We need to be more aggressive" because the disease continues to progress. Thus, a different drug is used or added, increasing the potential for withdrawal syndrome, side effects, or liver and kidney damage.

In any crime story, there is usually a hero (the protagonist), a villain (the perpetrator) and a victim. The victim is harassed by the perpetrator and in comes the hero to prevent further harm from being inflicted. This common plot occurs in everyday life too. A medical doctor can play hero or villain. One who performs a life saving surgery is a hero. But a medical doctor who tells a patient, "We need to be more aggressive" is a perpetrator. I highly recommend you avoid playing the role of the victim.

If your medical doctor suggests that you require another drug because he or she wants to be *a little* more aggressive in the treatment of your disease, turn around, walk away and look for a second opinion. The increased risk of withdrawal syndrome, side effects, liver damage and kidney damage are not worth it.

5

DRUG-INDUCED DISEASES

"Insanity: doing the same thing over and over again and expecting different results."

— Albert Einstein

The public generally does not believe that the almighty medical doctor could be the cause of a patient's disease — they are flawless in the detection of disease, omniscient in the realm of healthcare and will never do any harm. I, too, once believed this whimsical falsehood until I learned about doctor-induced diseases. One rainy day in the winter of 2002, this unimaginable concept entered my reality.

A nephrologist contacted me to pay his office a visit. I handed my business card to the receptionist and took a seat. As I waited, I wondered, "Why on earth does a kidney specialist want to speak with a pharmaceutical sales rep who sells anti-depressants? I'm supposed to sell to psychiatrists who treat depression." After a few minutes, the receptionist led me down the hallway to the doctor's office.

I greeted the doctor and we exchanged pleasantries. I noticed that he had been conducting a website search on his computer. All of a sudden multiple internet windows began popping up on his computer screen. Not knowing how to stop this, he kept clicking the "x" at the top right hand corner of each new window. However, as soon as he closed one box, another ten popped open. His face turned red as one popped open displaying voluptuous women in scanty lingerie. He continued for ten minutes until I could see fatigue setting in on his clicking finger. He could not win this pointless game no matter how quickly he clicked his mouse.

He must have clicked a link which caused new windows to proliferate like cells in an uncontrolled cancer. Ironically, he was attempting to use the clicking of the mouse, the original cause of the incessant pop-up windows, as his solution.

After fifteen minutes, he finally decided to reboot his computer, turned to me and said, "I just don't understand these things. These computers. Sometimes they create more problems than actual solutions."

As we waited for his computer to restart, he explained his interest in learning about the anti-depressant I promoted. Being a kidney specialist, the treatment of depression and other mood disorders was not exactly part of his specialty, so I asked, "Why are you interested in the treatment of Major Depressive Disorder?"

"One of my patients is taking a drug called Interferon for hepatitis and is beginning to experience depression as a side effect."

I immediately presented him the FDA clinical studies that proved my anti-depressant was effective for Major Depressive Disorder and requested his verbal commitment to prescribe the medication. I paused for a response. He agreed to prescribe it and I walked away satisfied. I had closed a deal like a well-trained pharmaceutical sales puppet.

On my drive home, I had an epiphany. If depression is one disease that can result from taking one drug, could other pharmaceuticals cause additional diseases? I struggled for minutes with this concept, like an atheist and agnostic debating the existence of God. I did not want it to exist. But the logical order of transpired events indicated that it was a true and very real phenomenon. I had learned about iatrogenesis.

Iatrogenesis is the formal name for *doctor-induced disease*. During the three month intensive training I received as a pharmaceutical sales rep, I had never heard the term. No one explained that the side effects of a pharmaceutical could actually present as a full-blown diagnosable disease. This type of information is intentionally concealed from pharmaceutical sales reps and the public.

I had been sheltered from learning the real dangers of pharmaceutical drugs. By lacking the word "iatrogenesis" in my vocabulary, the concept remained abstract. I did not know what to call it, nor if it was even true. Was it a figment of my own imagination, like identifying animals among the cloud formations in the sky?

My pharmaceutical sales colleagues and I were trained to be ignorant of drug-induced diseases. We were subliminally brainwashed into believing our products would save the world. After all, it is easier to sell a product that you believe in. The opposite is also true. If I knew what I carried in my sample bag had the potential to create or cause other diseases, I would have walked away from the industry altogether. Other than practitioners of euthanasia like Dr. Kevorkian, who sells a poison willingly?

But then I saw a light, and came to this simple realization: These drugs. Sometimes they create more problems than actual solutions.

DRUG-INDUCED DISEASES

The very first book to clearly catalogue and explain the phenomenon of *Drug-Induced Diseases* was written by L. Meyler and H.M. Peck in 1962. Before a scientific book is published, a significant amount of clinical data must be gathered. Therefore, allopathic medical doctors had known that pharmaceuticals cause diseases long before 1962.

Studies have documented the occurrence of drug-induced diseases since modern medicine began. The very first volume of *Drug-Induced Diseases* included nearly 200 pages of evidence. It underwent revisions and the fourth edition was published by 1968.

In 1964, two years after the first edition of *Drug-Induced Diseases* was published, Louis Lasagna revised the Hippocratic Oath. Was it mere coincidence that he removed the statement to avoid giving poisons to patients?

In the 1960s, allopathic medical doctors had the opportunity to make a moral decision to stop prescribing pharmaceuticals that cause withdrawal syndrome, side effects, liver damage, kidney failure and drug-induced diseases. Instead, they rewrote the sacred pledge all medical doctors make to society. Chapter One makes it clear that pharmaceutical drug therapies provide no realistic solutions to our society's health problems. Even more unthinkable, they may actually be contributing to it.

In 2005, two pharmacists published an updated version of the book called *Drug-Induced Diseases: Prevention, Detection, and Management.* The authors, James E. Tisdale and Douglas A. Miller, thoroughly detail in 870 pages the multiple conditions and diseases patients can actually develop from specific pharmaceuticals. Only five years later, the second edition bloated to 1,110 pages with the inclusion of additional documentation. We can only assume future editions will be even larger.

It is now well documented that:

- Lupus Erythematosus[44,45,46,47,48,49]
- Hypothyroidism[50,51,52,53,54,55,56,57,58,59]
- Leukemia[60,61,62,63,64,65]
- Lymphoma[66,67,68,69,70]
- Breast, endometrial, bladder, skin cancers[71,72,73,74,75,76]
- and many more diseases can all be drug-induced.

In 1962, allopathic medical doctors and the medical establishment chose to bury that data from the public. They hid it like a repressed memory in the darkest corner of pharmacy school libraries to collect dust and be ignored. Medical doctors failed to read it and now more patients have developed additional diseases. These books are available everywhere with just a few clicks by searching "drug-induced disease" on the web. Multiple sources list the dangers of psychiatric, cardiovascular, cancer and osteoporosis drugs, among others.

I have a friend who is a traditional naturopath and training as a Registered Nurse at the University of California, San Francisco. I was searching for a medical doctor in her network who was trained to identify diseases caused by pharmaceutical drugs. I establish referral partnerships with medical doctors to properly guide my nutritional clients off medications they no longer need.

I asked her, "Do you know of any medical doctors who are iatrogenesis specialists?"

She responded, "All of them. These doctors. Sometimes they create more problems than actual solutions."

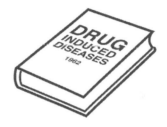

STANDING ON THE SIDELINES

In 2009, my uncle, a day trader, visited his Internist in Walnut Creek, CA for problems of low motivation and lethargy. His calls, puts and option trades were not going well, and he was concerned. The doctor diagnosed Major Depressive Disorder and prescribed an anti-depressant. My uncle had heard about the potential side effects from a television commercial. He had never taken any pharmaceuticals before because of the horror stories he heard from others at his office, including a coworker who developed ovarian cancer after taking chlomiphene to improve her chances of pregnancy and his senior manager who developed breast cancer from hormone replacement therapy.[77,78] So he asked his doctor, "Are there any side effects I should be on the lookout for? If I develop any of them, what should I do?"

His medical doctor responded, "Don't worry. This drug is safe. All pharmaceutical drugs are thoroughly tested before they are FDA approved for use on the prescription market. I trust the FDA. They manage the safety and quality of all pharmaceutical medications." My uncle remained skeptical, unsure that the FDA really does everything possible to protect us from harmful pharmaceutical products. He researched the FDA's level of scrutiny in testing and monitoring dangers after drugs are released to the general public.

He discovered a continuing education article entitled "Clinical, Therapeutic, and Recognition of Drug-Induced Disease" released in 1995 by Med Watch, founded in 1993 by the FDA for reporting adverse events, side effects or medical errors of pharmaceuticals and medical devices. It is well aware once the FDA approves a drug for prescription, potential for additional drug-induced diseases can arise.[79] See Figure 6.

If the FDA relies on the reporting of side effects after a drug has been approved, why should my uncle believe any drug is ever safe?

Nevertheless, not all allopathic medical doctors believe drug-induced diseases occur. In January 2012, I attended a dinner event at Skates on the Bay restaurant in Berkeley, CA with multiple medical doctors. I sat with a psychiatrist and an obstetrician. We engaged in normal conversation about our families and hobbies. They eventually shared with me the work they performed as medical

When a drug goes to market, we know everything about its safety.

Wrong.

1-800-FDA-1088.

FDA MEDWATCH
If it's serious, we need to know.

Figure 6. Image from a June 1995 MedWatch CE article.

doctors, then asked what I did for a living. I informed them that I was learning how to identify drug-induced diseases to help my nutritional clients understand the causes of their diseases. The psychiatrist was shocked. "Where are you learning about this? Is there a course somewhere?"

I cringed at the irony. Despite the MedWatch continuing education article, these two medical specialists had never heard of such a phenomenon. The day MedWatch or the FDA proactively brings national awareness of this issue to both the general public and all licensed medical doctors is the day the pharmaceutical industry loses credibility as the bearers of health. Currently, no educational institution endorses a formal curriculum for the identification and detection of drug-induced diseases. Medical schools do not dare teach this subject because intelligent medical students will realize that the pharmaceutical medicines they are trained to feed their patients are toxic and fail to restore wellness.

I responded to the psychiatrist, "I found a book on the internet called *Drug-Induced Diseases* and started correlating it with the nutritional clients that I've helped. The information offers my clients an explanation for their health conditions."

It is frightening that few medical doctors know that drug-induced diseases exist, for they are on the frontlines of prescribing pharmaceutical medications. One problem is that only 5-20% of iatrogenic events are ever reported, indicating that drug-induced diseases are drastically underestimated.[80,81,82] Their incidence may be significantly greater than the FDA, MedWatch and post-marketing agencies report to the public.

Allopathic medical doctors have the most power to perpetuate iatrogenesis — or prevent it. The second most powerful group is the public — each and every one of us. Fortunately, holistic health care practitioners nationwide know how to use specific tools to identify drug-induced diseases, restore patient health and reduce patient reliance on drugs with the help of their prescribing physician.

Question #5 to ask your allopathic medical doctor:
Is this pharmaceutical drug you are prescribing known to cause another disease?

SURGEON GENERAL'S WARNING

The Surgeon General requires cigarette manufacturers to place a warning on every cigarette package to educate consumers that smoking raises the risk of lung cancer, heart disease, emphysema and pregnancy complications.

An intelligent person would expect similar warnings on pharmaceutical products. Is it possible that the FDA and Med Watch are inundated with incoming reports of side effects or drug-induced diseases, but cannot find time to create such a label? Or maybe they are afraid the public will finally see through the smoke and mirrors of "healthcare" and realize that pharmaceutical medicine is a vehicle for continuous revenue growth and profit margins.

DRUG-INDUCED DEATH

Death is perhaps the worst drug-induced adverse event. It currently affects up to 98,000 people a year in the United States.[83] Nearly 270 people die every day due to taking pharmaceutical drugs. The annual number of deaths caused by Western medicine is an astounding 783,936 per year.[84] Evidently, the American medical system is the leading cause of death and injury in the US.

The International Statistical Classification of Diseases and Related Health Problems, 10th revision (ICD-10), is a medical classification list by the World Health Organization for the coding of signs, symptoms and causes of injury, disease and death. ICD-10 codes are often required to properly record the causes of drug-induced deaths.[85]

Hospitals, medical doctors and other medical professionals know pharmaceuticals have the ability to cause fatalities. Homicide is an act or instance of unlawfully killing another human being. Do medical doctors carry a badge or card of immunity that allows them to prescribe a deadly pharmaceutical and suffer no legal consequences?

Medical doctors are trained to believe newer pharmaceuticals are safer than older ones. Sadly, newer pharmaceuticals have a higher risk of withdrawal from the market. Since the 1950s, the FDA approved 52 medications which were later withdrawn due to unexpected deaths or organ failures. Twenty-eight (over half) of the 52 were withdrawn between 2000 to 2011, which means the approval of "mistake" drugs is occurring more often now than 50 years ago. (See Figure 7 for recent drug withdrawals.) It appears that the FDA's drug approval process is not designed to protect the consumer. Perhaps it is time to reconsider your trust in the FDA.

Pharmaceutical Name	Withdrawn	Reason for market withdrawal
Hydromorphone (Palladone®)	2005	Risk of overdose
Pemoline (Cylert®)	2005	Risk of liver damage
Ximelagatran (Exanta®)	2006	Risk of liver damage
Pergolide (Permax®)	2007	Risk of heart valve damage
Tegaserod (Zelnorm®)	2007	Causes heart attack & stroke
Aprotinin (Trasylol®)	2007	Risk of death
Lumiracoxib (Prexige®)	2008	Risk of liver damage
Rimonabant (Acomplia®)	2008	Risk of severe depression
Efalizumab (Raptiva®)	2009	Risk of leukoencephalopathy
Sibutramine (Meridia®)	2010	Risk of heart disease
Mylotarg®	2010	Lack of efficacy
Drotrecogin alfa (Xigris®)	2011	Lack of efficacy

Figure 7. Withdrawn drugs from 2005-2011.

In order for a pharmaceutical company to attain FDA approval to market and sell a drug, it must run clinical trials that prove a drug is both safe and effective.

This process is conducted in 3 phases:

- Phase 1 screens for the safety of the experimental drug. A drug is tested in a healthy population to examine the potential for organ damage, side effects and possible death.
- Phase 2 measures the experimental drug's "efficacy" in treating a sample of the intended patient population.
- Phase 3 compares for efficacy against a placebo (a sugar pill deemed to have no therapeutic benefit).

The FDA reviews studies for experimenter bias and tampering of data. Unfortunately, this process has many flaws and opportunities for doctoring the numbers. *Overdosed America, The Broken Promise of American Medicine* by Dr. John Abramsons is an excellent account by an honest and inquisitive medical doctor who looked deeply into clinical studies conducted by pharmaceutical companies. He found the original data and results from these studies were skewed to augment commercial profit. The FDA's system is not sufficiently equipped to fully protect the public.

The largest recall of pharmaceutical products occurred in 2004 with Vioxx®, estimated to have caused 25,000 to 55,000 deaths. Dr. David Graham, a whistle blower within Merck, the manufacturer of Vioxx®, testified before the United States Senate. He estimated that 88,000 to 139,000 Americans experienced heart attacks as a side effect from the drug with a 30-40% mortality rate. Vioxx®, at its height, was taken by over 20 million Americans.

When the news broke that Vioxx increased heart attacks, Merck's stock prices took a slight slap on the wrist, but business boomed on. Although Vioxx® was the most publicized drug recall, eighteen more drugs have been withdrawn since then.

Avandia®, or rosiglitazone, was found in Europe to be associated with increased risk of stroke, heart failure and mortality in patients over 65 and was pulled off the market there.[86] Yet it is still available in the U.S., despite the knowledge of these risks.

<u>**Question #6 to ask your allopathic medical doctor**</u>:
Is the pharmaceutical drug you are prescribing me known to cause death?

HUMAN GUINEA PIGS

Before my graduation ceremony at the Greek Theatre of U.C. Berkeley in 2001, I carried a camcorder and randomly interviewed many of my closest friends and classmates about their future after Berkeley. One aspired to volunteer for the Peace Corps to help people in underdeveloped nations. Another friend shared his dream to study acupuncture and learn to heal people with needles and herbs. I asked a third friend, "So, Rob, what plans do you have now that you've graduated with a biology degree from one of the most prominent public academic institutions?"

"Oh, I don't know. Maybe go find a job testing bulletproof vests. I heard the impact of shots to the chest will make my abs stronger." Though he was joking, people who are prescribed newly released pharmaceuticals are like bulletproof vest testers. Many die or experience serious organ damage prior to the FDA's removal of dangerous drugs from the market. It's up to you to ask yourself if you feel safe taking a new FDA approved drug? Are you willing to sacrifice your life to test the safety of a "new and improved" pharmaceutical drug product? Would you like to test whether your liver and kidney organs are capable of metabolizing and excreting a potentially harmful substance? If you plan on taking a newer medication, be sure your life insurance premium is paid for and your policy is active. You may be giving a precious gift to benefit someone down the road. My hope is that you turn around and look elsewhere to improve your health. I recommend you look up my friend who eventually learned how to heal others with acupuncture needles, herbs and whole food nutrition.

6

THE ILLUSION OF MEDICINE

"As a magician I promise never to reveal the secret of any illusion to a non-magician, unless that one swears to uphold the Magician's Oath in turn. I promise never to perform any illusion for any non-magician without first practicing the effect until I can perform it well enough to maintain the illusion of magic."

— The Magician's Oath

My friend Raymond is an amazing magician who performs at family events and friends' birthday parties. He considers himself an amateur, but he can awe five jaw-dropping friends the same way David Copperfield does on a stage in front of thousands. Raymond recently participated in a companywide talent show called Intel's Got Talent 2012. He began by pulling out a newspaper, just off the press, while bantering about how the media warns us the world is falling apart. "Our company's stock remains stagnant." He tore the paper in half and stacked the halves. "Banks cannot curtail the housing market downfall, and foreclosures are on the rise." He tore across the sheets once again. "Cruise ships are sinking in Europe." The newspaper was torn one last time. He then compacted the pieces into a crumpled ball. "A stagnant stock is better than a dropping stock. Houses are the cheapest ever. Vacation cruise trip packages are now less expensive due to tourist fears of drowning." He paused. "Which means it's time to cash out, go buy a house and book a cruise." Then he unraveled the ball to show the audience sheets of a whole newspaper, completely intact. The audience claps and screams in amazement. He has magically restored what was apparently a pile of torn newspaper fragments into a whole and completely fresh Sunday paper.

A good magic show tickles our ears, eyes, mind and heart in unison. You ask yourself, "How did the magician do that?" A magician understands how to trick the mind and fool the senses by gently guiding them with techniques of misdirection. To understand the magical elements we must be curious enough to learn a little about the art of misdirection. It's quite simple. Raymond read a few key books to study the tricks of the trade in a matter of hours.

The pharmaceutical industry uses its own sleight of hand. They manipulate advertisements for misdirection, creating the illusion that we require pharmaceutical products for health and wellness. A medical doctor convincing you that a drug is the magic bullet to end all your problems is an obvious case of misdirection. The cholesterol illusion is one that is most widely perpetuated.

THE CHOLESTEROL ILLUSION

Cholesterol lowering pharmaceuticals are referred to as statin drugs. The industry has misled the public into believing that proteins are the same as cholesterol. They are not. It inaccurately labels HDLs as "good" cholesterol and LDLs as "bad" cholesterol. Newsflash: HDL stands for High Density Lipoprotein and LDL stands for Low Density Lipoprotein. HDL and LDL are proteins, not cholesterol.

Cholesterol is a lipid, a fatty substance. Our bodies require cholesterol. HDLs simply transport cholesterol from the organs and tissues back to the liver to be converted into bile. Bile is required for proper fat digestion and assimilation of the essential fat-soluble vitamins A, D, E, K and F. LDLs transport the cholesterol from the liver to the tissues and endocrine glands such as the adrenals, testicles and ovaries. Cholesterol is *the* precursor material of many important hormones. A man's body cannot produce appropriate amounts of testosterone without sufficient levels of cholesterol, nor a woman's estrogen and progesterone without sufficient levels of cholesterol.

I have known Mike and Alice for seven years. Mike is a truck driver who is out on the road for weeks at a time transporting all sorts of freight in his big rig. He recently sent me his blood work results and I noticed that both his LDL and HDL levels were below healthy levels. I asked, "Have you been taking a statin drug?"

He confessed. "I've been taking these damn drugs for years. Now I have muscle pains and forget which roads I'm supposed to be on so my deliveries are delayed." Ten years ago, Mike was told by his medical doctor that he had high cholesterol.

I noticed Mike's testosterone levels were also low. His testicles could not produce testosterone due to a shortage of precursor material. His testicles wanted to get his hotrod going, but he was running out of gas. I informed him that he needed to have his medical doctor lower his dosage because his testicles were starving for cholesterol.

"But... why didn't my.... my medical doctor... um... tell me about the um... that the testicles needed cholesterol to make the um... the um... testosterone?"

Cholesterol is an essential building material of the brain and because Mike's body lacked a sufficient amount of it, his memory may have been negatively impacted. He paused between sentences as if his mind had parked at a rest stop to search for words. Alice mentioned that ever since he began taking the cholesterol lowering medications, his responsiveness and overall mental function had declined. "His moods have ups and downs, but I figured it was because he has a stressful job. Is cholesterol required for a balanced endocrine system?" I explained that for optimal health, our bodies require ample supplies of cholesterol for the production of many essential hormones, including cortisol, dehydroepiandrosterone, pregnenolone and aldosterone. The statin drugs have the potential to cause male and female hormonal imbalances.

We need to consider the functions of cholesterol, rather than fear it blindly. Cholesterol is a fatty substance predominantly created by the liver as a building block for all of the cells in our body. Cholesterol has many important functions:

- Cholesterol makes cell membranes waterproof to maintain biochemical balance inside and outside the cell.[87,88]

- Cholesterol is a repair substance, which is why it pervades scar tissue (including within arteries).[89]

- Cholesterol is a precursor to Vitamin D.[90]

- Cholesterol is a precursor to bile salts, vital for digestion and assimilation of fat-soluble vitamins.

- Cholesterol provides protection against cancer.[91]

- Cholesterol is vital to proper neurological function for memory.[92]

- Cholesterol assists with serotonin (5-HT) receptor function in brain.[93]

- Cholesterol is a major component of myelin sheaths lining nerve tissue and the brain.[94]

- Cholesterol protects against free radical damage that leads to heart disease and cancer.[95,96]

- Cholesterol is required for the production of steroid hormones, including testosterone, estrogen and progesterone.[97]

When I explained this to Mike, he asked, "So why are so many people taking drugs to lower cholesterol? My doctor has been prescribing it to me for ten years. Doesn't it prevent heart disease or heart attacks?"

I showed him the fine print in a 2004 magazine advertisement (I had saved) for Lipitor®, the highest grossing pharmaceutical and most commonly prescribed statin drug in the US.[98,99] "LIPITOR® has not been shown to prevent heart disease or heart attacks." See Figure 8. Mike and Alice were confused. Why would they lower their cholesterol levels if there was little to no cardiovascular benefit?

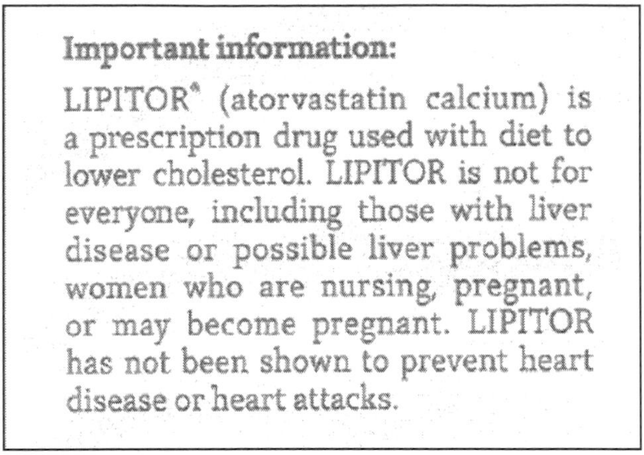

Important information:

LIPITOR® (atorvastatin calcium) is a prescription drug used with diet to lower cholesterol. LIPITOR is not for everyone, including those with liver disease or possible liver problems, women who are nursing, pregnant, or may become pregnant. LIPITOR has not been shown to prevent heart disease or heart attacks.

Figure 8. Fine print in a magazine advertisement.

Statin drugs are widely known to cause muscle pain, or myopathy.[100,101,102] Over 900 clinical studies document the side effects of statin drugs. [103] Furthermore, they have also been shown to increase the risk of developing type 2 diabetes and cancer.[104,105,106] I asked, "Did your doctor warn you about the dangers when he prescribed this medication?"

"No. But I'm damn sure as hell going to ask him why he didn't!" Mike was furious. I reminded him to stay calm and assured him that we will be able to get him well again. In fact, we needed his medical doctor to work with us, so I encouraged him not to burn any bridges. His job was to speak with his doctor about the best method to titrate off the medication. I also suggested he and Alice read *The Cholesterol Myth: Exposing the Fallacy That Saturated Fat and Cholesterol Cause Heart Disease* by Uffe Ravnskov because it provides much more information on the statin drugs than I have shared in just a few paragraphs.

Over the course of three months, through nutritional upgrades and a collaborative effort with his doctor, we were able to help Mike raise his cholesterol to a healthy level, restore healthy testosterone levels without the use of hormone replacement therapy, sharpen his memory and resolve his muscle pain. He's improved his work efficiency 300% and not made a late delivery since.

SPIN SELLING

Prior to my first interview with a pharmaceutical sales manager, an executive headhunter mentioned to me that drug companies focus primarily on candidates with a strong track record for closing sales. Even though I believed my degrees in molecular and cell biology and psychology would benefit my competence as a pharmaceutical sales representative, she reminded me to highlight my selling strengths during interviews.

After I was hired, I learned that the interview process included a particular exercise to weed out incompetent candidates and grant a rite of passage for those who had the potential to flourish as a pharmaceutical sales rep. I had to conduct a mock sales pitch to the hiring manager, who assumed the role of a doctor. I was provided only one fact about the mock drug: it invariably led to an adverse reaction so intolerable that 7% of patients would stop the medication.

I presented its features and benefits, and I strategically added, "Ninety-three percent of all your patients will receive benefit from the drug with no complications whatsoever. That means, doctor, it will be easy for you to prescribe and your patients will maintain a high rate of compliance."

That one statement sealed the job for me. I proved I could manipulate the intention of data with a creative use of language to create the illusion that any doctor could prescribe it for life with few complaints. This is referred to as spin selling — the ability to hide the weakness of a product and bring focus on the positive benefits the target buyer is interested in hearing. Pharmaceutical reps and allopathic doctors are masters of spin.

When I was thirteen years old, I joined a seven-day, 50-mile hike near Mount Whitney with my Boy Scout troop. We hiked in extreme heat and did not shower for days. Hungry mosquitoes hovered around us, waiting to swarm in for a quick all you can drink buffet. Tempers were short among our group of boys who wanted to be home playing video games in the comfort of air conditioned family rooms. One boy accidentally tripped another, generating a nasty comment. A dialogue of insults ensued. One of the hike leaders yelled out, "Hey! If you don't have anything nice to say, don't say anything at all."

I turned to my younger brother. "Hey, little brother, you smell better than chicken manure today." We both laughed because our four days of accumulated body odor didn't bother us anymore. I didn't know it back then, but I was practicing the art of spin selling in preparation for my role as a pharmaceutical sales representative.

TREAT THE PERSON, NOT THE NUMBER

The Rule of Threes is an important guide for prioritizing the basic needs to preserve and maintain human life. Without air for three minutes, our brain shuts down due to lack of oxygen. Without water for three days, out body enters shock. Without food for three weeks, our tissues and organs run out of nutrients to enable bodily functions. Clean air, pristine water and nutrient dense foods are essential components of our lives. I have yet to meet someone who can live without drinking water. Ironically, the pharmaceutical industry has convinced many allopathic medical doctors that water is the cause of high blood pressure.

The easiest, but most dangerous, way to lower blood pressure is to decrease blood volume. Most of the water in our body is in the plasma of the blood, which is composed of 93% water and 7% other substances (proteins, glucose, mineral ions, hormones, etc.) By decreasing the volume of blood, blood pressure will also drop.

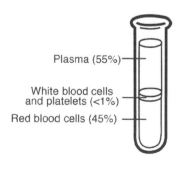

Plasma (55%)

White blood cells and platelets (<1%)

Red blood cells (45%)

Medical doctors often prescribe diuretics which mandate the adrenal and kidney organs to decrease the water volume in blood. By inducing increased urination frequency and volume, diuretic medications lower blood pressure. Doctors merely focus on decreasing a number, while ignoring the Rule of Threes. Thus, many are quick to prescribe a diuretic, but neglect to investigate the cause of high blood pressure.

To see if you are dehydrated, note which symptoms you have that may be due to the loss of water from your body:

2% total fluid loss	5% total fluid loss	10% total fluid loss
• Thirst	• Increased pulse	• Muscle spasms
• Loss of appetite	• Increased respiration	• Vomiting
• Dry skin	• Decreased sweating	• Racing pulse
• Skin flushing	• Increased body temperature	• Shriveled skin
• Dark colored urine	• Extreme fatigue	• Dim vision
• Dry mouth	• Muscle cramps	• Painful urination
• Fatigue or weakness	• Headaches	• Confusion
• Chills	• Nausea	• Difficulty breathing
• Head rushes	• Tingling of the limbs	• Seizures
		• Chest or abdominal pain
		• Unconsciousness

A holistic health care practitioner understands that high blood pressure may be a symptom of multiple organs becoming fatigued or undernourished. The liver, large intestine, bone, lungs, skin, kidneys, adrenal, thyroid, pituitary and hypothalamus glands all play a part in regulating blood pressure to ensure your blood, the medium through which all nutrients and oxygen are carried to and from various tissues, reaches every cell of your body. Since water in the blood carries nutrients and oxygen to every cell and organ of the body, it is an essential substance for optimal health and wellness. I highly recommend *Your Body's Many Cries for Water* by F. Batmanghelidj, MD to understand the importance of water for the human body. Water is NOT the cause of high blood pressure.

Question #7 to ask your allopathic medical doctor:
For any health issue or out of range lab value, ask: Which organs need help and what can you do to regenerate them?

DIALYSIS PROVIDES LITTLE HOPE

Though the dialysis machine may be one of the greatest inventions created by NASA, modern technologies can never fully replace what nature provides us. Dialysis replaces only 10% of normal renal (kidney) function, so patients remain in a permanently toxic state. Moreover, dialysis tubing is known to leach toxic chemicals into a patient's blood.[107] These chemicals, infection from the treatment process and low blood pressure all shorten life expectancy.

The life expectancy for patients who undergo dialysis drops significantly. When a nephrologist recommends dialysis to any patient showing signs of failing kidneys, the recommendation is not a solution to address the causes, but rather a prognosis — the likely outcome is death (see Figure 9). If you know someone who has been told their kidneys are failing, I highly recommend a visit to someone like Dr. Nancy (see Case Study on next page) who helped John and many more patients restore optimal kidney function and avoid dialysis.

Patient Age	Non-diabetic	Diabetic
20 to 39	20 years	8 years
40 to 59	13 years	8 years
60 to 74	7 years	5 years

Source: Handbook of Kidney Transplantation by Gabriel M Danovitch.

Figure 9. Life expectancy for patients on dialysis treatment.

THE MYTH OF EXCELLENCE

Malena is a 31 year old woman of Cambodian descent who was diagnosed with rheumatoid arthritis seven years ago. Most of her joints continued to ache despite taking prednisone for inflammation and methotrexate to suppress her immune system. Her primary care physician originally told her the cause of her disease was unknown. As an autoimmune disease, he explained, her immune system was attacking her own body's tissues.

Case Study – Preventing Kidney Failure

Dr. Nancy is a colleague and a Doctor of Chiropractic. John is a patient of hers, who was taking seven medications, five of which were to lower his blood pressure which was diagnosed over ten years ago. He was told by a nephrologist that his kidneys showed signs of failing. "There is nothing we can do. My professional recommendation is that you go on dialysis." John knew the quality of life on dialysis would be depressing, so looked elsewhere for solutions.

Dr. Nancy informed him that his blood pressure lowering drugs were overworking his kidneys by forcing them to excrete more water than normal, even though his body needed more water. He was severely dehydrated from taking a diuretic and other blood pressure lowering medications for many years. His symptoms were in the 2% and 5% range for loss of total body fluid. His body was thirsty. Using epocrates.com, she showed him the additional stress on his medications contributed to his kidneys.

Furosemide: 88% excreted through the kidneys
Amlodipine: 60% excreted through the kidneys
Hydralazine: Kidneys excrete 90%
Carvedilol: 16% excreted through the kidneys
Aspirin: Mainly excreted through the kidneys
Zemplar: 16-18% excreted through the kidneys
Clonidine: 40-60% excreted through the urine

She also pointed out that three of his medications have been linked to interstitial nephritis (inflammation of the kidneys), which may lead to chronic or permanent kidney damage. [108],[109],[110],[111] Dr. Nancy guided him through a three-week detoxification program. He lost sixteen pounds of excess fat tissue, upgraded his eating habits and received nutritional and chiropractic care on a regular basis. His kidneys showed signs of regeneration in as little as one month, and his blood pressure normalized. She then partnered with a medical doctor to guide John off the medications he no longer needed. John is feeling vibrant and energetic about living life again. His kidneys are fully functional and dialysis is no longer a consideration.

Six months before Malena came to see me, her medical doctor had told her that her disease was progressing and he needed to take more aggressive measures. She was scared because the prednisone was already weakening her bones and making her skin thinner, whereas the methotrexate made her more susceptible to infections. She fell sick with a debilitating cold every other month, leaving her incapable of going to work. Her colleagues no longer relied on her for important projects with strict deadlines. She had lost hope and was filled with fear.

I told her, "The body has an amazing ability to heal. Your immune system is part of who you are, and we need it to be strong enough to prevent you from becoming sick and missing work." Besides desiring a successful career, she also wanted to contribute to society by volunteering at local charities and donating blood.

Malena and I worked together for two months to upgrade her diet, strengthen her immune system and decrease her antibodies. Once we saw that the autoimmune component was resolved, she visited her medical doctor who guided her off the methotrexate. Within another eight months, Malena no longer suffered from joint pain and lives completely medication free. She now leads a team of six coworkers, donates blood regularly and travels once a year to Cambodia to volunteer for an organization that sponsors orphans for formal education.

Allopathic medical doctors have few tools to restore optimal wellness, health and vitality. Unfortunately, they also confuse patients by diagnosing them with 'incurable,' 'progressing' or 'idiopathic' (no known cause) diseases. Telling Malena that her disease was 'idiopathic' implied that he did not know how to help her heal. By 'incurable', he meant that he could not help, and he might make her situation worse. That her disease was 'progressing' meant he had made it worse or neglected to improve her health.

As a child watching the film *The Wizard of Oz* (1939), I believed the Wizard had the power to help Dorothy return home to Kansas. However, once we go behind the curtains and discover what is underneath the white coat, it is evident that the Wizard and Malena's doctor are merely ordinary people, just like you and me. As a child, I loved to watch the greatest magic shows of all. Today, many people pay for these performances with their medical co-pays.

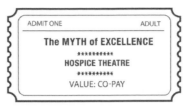

7

SALES & MARKETING GURUS

"Every doctor has his price."

— Any drug rep

Pharmaceutical companies are, perhaps, the best sales and marketing firms — better than the great branding companies like Ogilvy and Mather or The Coca-Cola Company. They have the ability to convince a whole population to consume toxic chemicals long-term and thereby expect health and wellness. They have set the bar high for anybody else to convince us otherwise.

Their marketing efforts are so pervasive and intrusive that people are extremely willing to follow their doctor's orders despite the fact that pharmaceuticals destroy livers and kidneys, lead to drug-induced diseases and even cause death. We are constantly bombarded by television commercials and magazine ads. Every doctor's visit exposes us to even more advertising to keep us believing the illusion of medicine. So how do they do it?

The first approach is to advertise directly to the consumer. The United States and New Zealand are the only two countries that permit advertising pharmaceuticals directly to consumers. Pharmaceutical companies argue that the public should not be denied access to the knowledge and awareness of conditions that could affect their health.

It's unfortunate that the patient-doctor relationship is compromised because patients can speak to their medical doctors about drugs they learned about from a television commercial. While marketing efforts appear to inform the public about important health issues, the real purpose is for commercial interests. By 1999, the average American was exposed to nine prescription drug advertisements on television every day. These are typically aired during prime time, shortly after dinner.

The same year, a Prevention magazine survey found that 80 percent of all patients said that they obtained a prescription for an advertised medicine when they requested it. What that means is the ads are creating the demand for prescription drugs and only 20 percent of medical doctors are saying no. Unfortunately, these ads are destroying the integrity of the medical doctor channel. Originally doctors were in charge of their patients' health and chose the proper treatment regimen — not the other way around. After all, they spent hundreds of thousands of dollars on their medical school tuition.

As direct consumer advertising took hold of the market, the drug industry profit margins skyrocketed from about 12% of research and development expenses in 1991 to 18% in 2001, while the rest of the Fortune 500 industries averaged 5% or less.[112] Figure 10, shows Direct To Consumer Advertising (DTCA) has risen each year.

PHARMACEUTICAL SELLING

Love and Other Drugs, a film featuring Anne Hathaway and Jake Gyllenhaal, provides an amusing depiction of pharmaceutical sales reps. The first 20 minutes of this movie provide an unbelievably accurate portrayal on how I, along with my storm trooper drug representative colleagues, literally invaded doctors' offices from the 1980s through 2002.

| Year | Spending (in billions) | |
	On DTC Advertising	On promotion to physicians
1997	$1.10	$3.90
1998	$1.30	$4.60
1999	$1.80	$4.80
2000	$2.50	$5.60
2001	$2.70	$5.90
2002	$2.60	$6.60
2003	$3.30	$7.40
2004	$4.00	$7.80
2005	$4.20	$7.20
Average annual percentage increase	19.6%	9%
Total percentage increase, 1997-2005	296.4%	86%

Source: U.S. Government Accountability Office

Figure 10. Annual spending on Direct to Consumer Advertising (DTCA) and spending on promotion to physicians during 1997-2005.

Drug representatives were allowed to invite medical doctors to musicals, sporting events and expensive dinners, all on the company dime. Many of the more aggressive drug reps would even purchase season passes to sporting events.

Pharmaceutical companies are known to have flown many medical doctors to Rome and other international travel destinations for two-week, all expenses paid vacations. In order to earn the trip, the doctor must achieve the status of highest prescriber for a particular drug. It makes me wonder what the difference is between an expensive gift and a bribe.

I entered the pharmaceutical industry in the year 2001. In early 2002, Pharmaceutical Research and Manufacturers of America (PhRMA) passed new guidelines to prevent drug reps from engaging in extravagant entertainment, bribes and lavish gifts. Needless to say, medical doctors were saddened, though loopholes existed since PhRMA is a collective establishment of all the major pharmaceutical companies. It makes me wonder if there is any irony that pharmaceutical companies manage the 3rd party organization responsible for regulating the ethics of their own sales and marketing practices.

From 2002 to 2006, I was allowed to provide medical doctors educational meals to present clinical data specific to the drugs I promoted. Technically, I was supposed to provide information regarding specific indications, safety profiles, drug-to-drug interactions and potential for withdrawal syndrome. I spent an average of $5,000 monthly, catering lunches to doctors' offices and hosting dinners at 5-star restaurants for doctors and their significant others. When I asked my manager what my monthly budget limit was, her words were, "Spend until I tell you to stop." She knew the more meals I scheduled with doctors, the more my drug would be prescribed.

I was never told to stop, even after spending $10,000 one month. We ordered bottles of wine that exceeded $200 each, ate full course meals, and tasted novel desserts as grand finales to evenings of superficial rapport and witty banter. If the doctor had a pet dog, he ordered the organic, pasture raised pork chop to go.

Despite the benefits, the pressures to meet sales goals were very high, requiring me to engage in a certain level of activity that was known to directly increase sales.

My company paid $500 honorariums to doctors allowing me to shadow them for a few hours, also referred to as a preceptorship. It was an opportunity to learn how that doctor conducted patient care, which allowed me to learn how to serve him or her as a better resource. These preceptorships were really an opportunity to hold a particular doctor accountable to prescribing the drugs I promoted. When a patient presented all the symptoms of Major Depressive Disorder, the doctor felt cornered to prescribe the antidepressant I promoted with me standing next to him. After all, I had arranged for him to receive a $500 honorarium. In my seven preceptorships, every doctor prescribed the drugs I promoted. Preceptorship honorariums were a great tool to guide a medical doctor into developing a new habit that increased my overall sales.

If you ever see a pharmaceutical sales rep in the patient room or your doctor's office, be aware that the prescription you received may have been influenced by him or her.

In addition to preceptorships, I also employed a different sales tactic for the medical doctors who were influential among their colleagues as "thought leaders" or "key opinion leaders." I identified six doctors in my sales territory to speak on behalf of the products I represented. Medical doctors know this can earn them additional revenues, and possibly trips to conventions with travel expenses reimbursed. The grant or honorarium for speaking one hour ranged from $500 to $5000.

Speaker candidates were usually high prescribers who already had extensive experience with the drug and could share with other doctors about their positive experiences. National pharmacy chains collect data detailing the prescribing habits of all doctors. These are sold to the pharmaceutical companies which distribute them weekly to their sales reps, creating competitive advantage over competitors. Since recruiting and training a doctor to become a speaker is a rather large investment, the data also allows drug reps to identify which doctors will provide the largest return on investment.

I worked with one doctor in Fremont, CA who was a horrible lecturer, lacking both charisma and proper hygiene. However, his potential to prescribe was at the top of my list. All my competitors were taking him to dinners at high-end restaurants. In order to be competitive, I trained him to become a speaker. I gave him a pedestal higher than the other drug reps could ever put him on. As soon as he was trained, I strategically set up a dinner for him to speak in front of his closest friends for thirty minutes. By inviting only his closest friends, I hedged any damaging effects his poor lecturing abilities could incur. At the end of the evening, he had the chance to catch up with his old friends from medical school. All attendees enjoyed a delicious meal that averaged $150 per person plus wine. My employer issued the doctor a check for $1,500 the following week, and my market share increased.

It was my job to ensure that all doctors exclusively prescribe my company's drugs. I literally raided doctors' offices and passed out all sorts of trinkets, booklets, notepads, pamphlets, pens, clipboards, clocks and umbrellas screaming, "Prescribe me!" Doctors knew I was there to implement the most effective marketing and sales tactics possible.

One day, I arranged a fifteen minute meeting with an Internal Medicine doctor who was one of my larger prescribers. Our conversation was very short, but it confirmed our agreement for me to cater lunch for his staff of forty once a week. In return, he would prescribe my drug exclusively when patients with Major Depressive Disorder walked into his clinic. I checked with my manager for an update on my entertainment spending limit. Again, she reiterated "Spend until I tell you to stop." The next day, I called the doctor to ask if he wanted his filet mignon rare or medium rare. This agreement increased my sales by 60%.

To be clear, not every medical doctor can be bought this easily. In fact, many of them are firm that their opinions about pharmaceuticals and scientific evidence are not compromised by drug reps. Yet, a review of doctor-to-drug company interactions published in The Journal of the American Medicine Association (JAMA) showed that these interactions have a mostly negative effect on the quality of medical care. Furthermore, it found the more interaction with the marketing personnel of pharmaceutical companies, the more likely that doctors would prescribe the newer, patented and more expensive drugs.

Cha-ching.

NOWHERE TO HIDE

Many of the pharmaceutical sales representatives that are hired have neither medical training nor a degree in the life sciences. Rather, they have top sales abilities and negotiation skills. Many sales reps can be very aggressive and are quite capable of selling gasoline to a person who has no car or pharmaceuticals to a person who has no illness. The intensity with which they operate is why some doctors prefer to not learn about newer pharmaceutical medicines from sales representatives. Instead, they receive new clinical information by attending Continuing Medical Education (CME) lectures.

Unfortunately, while they refrain from engaging in the wine-and-dine game, the CME lectures and seminars they attend are often sponsored and arranged by pharmaceutical sales representatives. I may have not had the chance to work the front office and detail these so-called "hard to reach" doctors, but I guarantee you that I was behind the scenes of many CME lectures at the local hospital continuing medical education lectures (also referred to as grand rounds).

I organized a CME lecture at one hospital that covered difficult to treat mood disorders, arranging for one of the company's more outstanding speakers from Stanford University. Technically, sales representatives were not allowed in the lecture hall; however, we were allowed to sponsor speakers and pay for their honorariums ($2000 in the case for the Stanford University medical professor's one hour lecture). During the lecture, I remained off the premises in order to allow the hospital staff to operate the event. At the end, I greeted the attendees as they exited. When I saw one of my "hard to reach" doctors walking out the door, I waved and attempted to speak with him. He quickly turned and scurried in the opposite direction. I let him flee because he just sat through an hour-long advertisement for the products I promoted. *You can run, but you can't hide.*

In many states, medical doctors are required to attend as many as 50 hours of CME seminars every year to maintain an active license to practice, and to be current with the facts and risks of the pharmaceuticals they are prescribing. However, pharmaceutical companies fund nearly 60% of doctors' continuing education.[113] In 2009, the pharmaceutical industry spent almost $1.2 billion on continuing medical education.[114] It is estimated that for every dollar the pharmaceutical industry invests in lectures and seminars, it earns $3.56 in increased sales — a great return on investment. [115] Pharmaceutical companies are able to penetrate every nook and cranny with some form of marketing, so doctors have nowhere to run and no place to hide.

PEER PRESSURE

In my seventh grade biology class, a classmate told me he wanted to become a medical doctor. I didn't really care. I was more fascinated with our pet mountain king snake which could swallow an entire mouse in one gulp.

The following week, that boy smashed a car window with a rock. Our principal caught him and his parents were not happy to hear that their son engaged in inappropriate behavior. They asked him why he did it. "I know it was wrong to break the window, but I was tricked into doing it by Bobby." His parents adored him and truly believed that their perfect angel must be telling the truth and let the issue go.

A few weeks later, he was caught again stealing DVD's from a local Target. Again 'Bobby' had coerced him. The parents felt they needed to speak with Bobby's parents, but were too busy to reach out and initiate contact. The boy then spray-painted graffiti on a school building and was put in detention. Is 'Bobby' the problem anymore? The same confusion exists in our current health care system.

In looking over the prescribing data, I once saw that one of my highest volume doctors had not been prescribing enough for me to earn my quarterly bonus, despite hosting him and his wife at expensive dinners on a regular basis and presenting the clinical data like a good drug rep. One evening, when his wife had gone to the powder room I asked him, "So doc, how else can I be a resource to you?"

"I would love to speak on behalf of your product and share the information with other medical doctors." He was a very eloquent and presentable individual with the charisma of Johnny Depp and with the suave style of the Dos Equis guy who tells us to "Stay thirsty, my friends." Who wouldn't want him to speak on behalf of their company?

"Consider it done. I'll register you to fly for a speaker training in New York, all expenses paid. Which weekend would your wife like to take a vacation to the Big Apple?"

After I arranged for him to be trained as a speaker, I found out that he spoke for all my competitors' companies. This tarnished reputation prevented him from influencing others. Everyone knew he gave lip service to whoever footed the bill and while he received a $2,000 honorarium per one-hour lecture given. Many of my doctors no longer found him a credible resource.

Strategically, I set up specific talks for him to give to insignificant groups of low volume prescribers. He earned an additional $8,000 a year because I arranged quarterly talks for him. Influencing his audiences was not my intention, but capturing every prescription that came from his office was. The highest prescribers have higher price tags. Even though medical doctors are very intelligent people, they occasionally enjoy being tricked by 'Bobby' into doing things they suspect might be wrong.

<u>Question #8 to ask your allopathic medical doctor</u>:
Have you ever been bought out? Let me rephrase that, have you ever gone out for dinner with a pharmaceutical sales representative and allowed them to foot the bill?

8

REVISIONING LIFE AND HEALTH

*"The only way to deal with an unfree world is to become so
absolutely free that your very existence is an act of rebellion."*

— Albert Camus

After five years, I finally left the pharmaceutical industry in 2006. I
felt I had sold my soul to the devil to earn a dollar. I even had all
sense of morality stripped from me. I had played the role of a sales
puppet to an industry that creates more health problems than
solutions.

In Chinese there is a saying, 職業病 (zhíyèbìng). It literally
translates into "disease of one's profession." I spent the next few
years in another country pursuing higher education and learning more
about different cultures, languages and holistic healing modalities
such as Traditional Chinese Medicine, Acupuncture, Tuina,
Chiropractic, Ayurveda, Reiki, Qigong, Reconnective Healing,
meditation, whole food nutrition, detoxification and more. Initially, I
experienced withdrawal from letting go of expensive meals, a
company car and quarterly bonuses. But the first step in healing from

the disease of my profession required me to find another life path, revise my career and redefine my vision of health.

When a ship is sinking, we all want to be the captain who saved the lives of others first. I urge you to lead by example. The ship will sink with you on it or not. The decisions you make today to improve your health will be noticed by many. Your skin will be clearer, your body will be fitter and your energy will return to the level of your early teens. As others notice, you will share with them the lifestyle changes you have made and they too will follow in your footsteps. You are not alone. I left the sinking ship in 2006 and now I work alongside thousands of holistic health care practitioners to help others do the same.

AN APOLOGY

I apologize to anybody who is taking a pharmaceutical drug that is a result of my previous promotional efforts. More importantly, I would like to wholeheartedly share a message with you (and anybody you know who is taking a pharmaceutical as 'medicine'): we all require whole and nutrient-dense foods (and not toxic chemicals) for nutrition. The rest of the book is a starting point from that perspective.

I ask all holistic health care practitioners to continue to help undo the karma I built. I am and forever will be grateful. I ask all medical doctors to offer your patients proper guidance to come off unnecessary pharmaceutical drugs as you begin to incorporate other holistic healing modalities in your practice.

SEEK OUT THE RIGHT DOCTOR

A 2002 survey with over 12,000 primary care physicians in the U.S. found that 66% of them were less than satisfied with the practice of medicine. Sixty percent said they would not recommend medicine as a career to others. Approximately one-third of the respondents said they planned to stop seeing patients in the next 1 to 3 years, and another 14% plan to cut back on patient care to part-time. Related to this lack of job satisfaction, medical doctors also suffer from the highest rate of suicide among professionals.[116]

More holistic medical doctors are in the making. Some of them have begun their journey to become holistic by calling themselves "minimalists," meaning they prefer to prescribe fewer pharmaceutical medications to avoid further complications. Minimalists are also experienced at guiding patients off pharmaceuticals in order to avoid withdrawal syndrome. They are one of the true partners for wellness.

A holistic health care practitioner is one who implements modalities that support the natural healing abilities of the body. The body only wants to do one thing when it is injured or plagued with illness — to heal. Holistic health care practitioners understand how the body does this and can help you in miraculous ways. Begin your search for one by asking your friends and family members for recommendations. Ask them, "Who is your acupuncturist? Who is your chiropractor? Who is your nutritionist?" The quest begins here and now.

MÜNCHAUSEN SYNDROME BY PROXY

The Sixth Sense is a film about a boy who could communicate with "dead people," the spirits of those who have passed on. Throughout the movie, he struggles to learn why spirits seek him at night and is constantly frightened by their unexpected appearances. At the end of the movie, he realizes that the spirits who visit him wish to relay a message to loved ones who still live in the physical world.

One day the boy attends the reception following a funeral of a nine year old girl who recently died. The spirit of the girl follows him into a room. At first he is frightened because he sees her vomit. When she recovers, she tells him a message. He walks over to the girl's grieving father and pulls out a video tape. "Your daughter wanted you to have this."

The father places the tape into a VCR and hits play. It is a recording of his little daughter in bed. The father smiles and is happy to see his daughter animated with life. After a few minutes, the mother of the girl enters with breakfast. The camcorder had captured the girl's mother adding a spoonful of poison to the girl's breakfast. The father's face erupts in horror and disgust seeing that his daughter died from daily dosing with poison. The spirit of the girl wanted to protect her younger sister from her mother and prevent her from facing the same ill fate that she did.

Münchausen Syndrome by Proxy is a pattern of behavior in which a caregiver deliberately exaggerates, fabricates or induces physical, psychological, behavioral or mental health problems in others. It is typically a parent, usually a mother, who intentionally causes illness in her child.

When a mother feeds her child a low-dose poison to induce illness, a medical doctor diagnoses her with Münchausen Syndrome by Proxy. When the pharmaceutical industry feeds our society poisons, what do we call that?

More importantly, what do you do to take control of your health?

Question #9 to ask your allopathic medical doctor:
If a medical doctor prescribes a poison for a child (or adult), who can diagnose him or her with Münchausen Syndrome by Proxy?

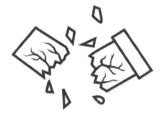

PART II:

FOOD AS MEDICINE

Luke Skywalker: *"I can't believe it."*

Yoda: *"That is why you fail."*

9

THE PERFECT DIET

"Tell me what you eat and I will tell you what you are."

— Anthelme Brillat-Savarin

When I first opened my nutritional practice, I asked every new client, "How is your diet?" The typical answer was, "It's pretty good. It could be better." What exactly does 'pretty good' mean? Is it good enough to prevent disease? Is it good enough so you never have to be concerned with your health?

In order to acquire real dietary information from my clients, I began to ask more specific questions. "What foods did you eat for breakfast?" The most common response from nearly every client does not include coffee, donuts, cereal or a pastry. It begins with a disclaimer, "Well… Today is not a typical day…"

Such a simple question warrants a simple recall of what one ate just a few hours earlier, but instead can elicit self-consciousness and the urge to justify poor eating habits. After they recite the foods they ate for breakfast, I ask about dinner. "Well, last night was not a typical evening…" What an interesting coincidence. Naturally, I follow up with, "what do you eat on a typical day?"

From their facial expression, I see the internal deliberation taking place. They don't want to come out and admit they applied margarine to their toast, because they know margarine is composed of trans fats (trans-fatty acid). Nor do they want to confess it was butter because they know butter contains saturated fat, which the public has incorrectly been taught to be harmful.[§] The mere struggle to provide the correct answer — the healthier of the two perceived evils — is one example where nutritional contradictions have left the general public confused.

Eventually, the inability to distinguish a healthy food from an unhealthy one pushes many individuals to forego eating habits based on health, choosing instead flavors that satisfy the palate. That most clients have little idea what their typical meal is indicates that current information about healthy eating lacks clarity. Should I eat fast food or not? Should I eat organic? Should I drink diet soda? Should I eat meat or only vegetables? Why is there so much confusion around the topic of nutrition? To correctly answer these questions, we must understand the history of food guidelines.

The United States Department of Agriculture (USDA) regularly releases updated dietary guidelines. Dr. Wilbur Atwater published the first nutrition guideline in 1894. In 1916, the guidelines were revised into five food groups called "Food for Young Children." During World War II, the USDA revised the guidelines to maintain nutritional standards under wartime food rationing.[117] Figure 11 is an announcement of the "Basic Seven" Food Groups diet, published in *The Free Lance-Star* on April 2, 1943 in Fredericksburg, Virginia at a time when margarine consumption was encouraged due to the shortage of butter.

During the 1940s, butter was considered a health food, while the health dangers of consuming margarine and other trans fat products

---

[§] In pages 169-170 of the book *Deep Nutrition: Why Your Genes Need Traditional Food*, author Catherine Shanahan, MD details how Ancel Keys confirmed trans fat, not saturated fat, leads to increased cardiovascular disease.

were not yet made public or even known. Consumers knew that margarine was and still is a commercially manufactured product. It is naturally gray, so in order to make it resemble butter, a yellow dye has to be added. Most manufacturers supplied yellow food-coloring capsules to consumers who could knead it into the margarine before serving. What would you do if a friend invited you over and asked you to prepare the margarine by mixing artificial food coloring into a bowl of a gray petroleum-looking substance to spread on your toast and corn?

Many of today's processed foods contain the yellow food dye, FD&C Yellow No. 5 which is known to contain benzidine, a Group 1 carcinogen by International Agency of Research on Cancer. [118], [119] Additionally, margarine and other processed food products containing trans fats are presently known to cause coronary heart disease, Alzheimer's, prostate cancer, insulin resistance and female infertility. [120],[121],[122],[123],[124] Perhaps the phony version of a real food is not always the safest.

> **To Demonstrate "Basic Seven" Diet**
>
> WASHINGTON, April 2.(P)—Wartime food demonstrations, aimed at maintaining nutrition standards, will be held soon all over the country.
>
> Under the slogan, "eat the basic 7 every day," the Agriculture Department suggested today in that connection that seven basic food groups which should be included in everyone's daily diet.
>
> They are: green and yellow vegetables; oranges, tomatoes, grapefruit (or raw cabbages or salad greens); potatoes and other vegetables and fruits; milk and milk products (such as cheese); meat, poultry, fish or eggs (or dried beans, peas, nuts or peanut butter); flour and cereals; and butter or fortified margarine (vitamin A added.).

Figure 11. Newspaper announcement of government food guidelines in 1943.

In 1956, the USDA shrank the "Basic Seven" into the "Basic Four" — vegetables, dairy, meats and grains. In 1992, they developed the "Food Pyramid" as an attempt to add recommended servings of each food group. Six to 11 servings of bread, cereal, rice and pasta occupy the base of the pyramid. Progressing up the Food Pyramid are vegetables, fruits, dairy, meats, fats, oils and sweets in lesser amounts. Unfortunately, the nationwide educational effort to publicize the 1992 Food Pyramid has left many impressionable adults and children to believe that grains, starches and cereals must be included in every meal if they represent the foundational layer of a government agency's food recommendation.

Since the Food Pyramid was first published in 1992, the Centers for Disease Control (CDC) has closely monitored the rates of obesity, which have consistently grown each year. The CDC website reports:

> "During the past 20 years, there has been a dramatic increase in obesity in the United States and rates remain high. More than one-third of U.S. adults (35.7%) and approximately 17% (or 12.5 million) of children and adolescents aged 2—19 years are obese."
>
> ~Center for Disease Control, 2012

It has been well studied and documented that a diet filled with grains and starches, which the body converts into sugar, is known to lead to blood sugar related disorders. *Good Calories, Bad Calories* by Gary Taubes provides a thorough scientific look into the potential health dangers from consumption of a diet high in refined grains, starches and sugars.

Observing poor health trends directly correlated to governmental nutritional recommendations, the USDA launched the MyPyramid campaign in 2005. It replaced the hierarchical levels of the Food Guide Pyramid with vertical wedges of different colors in a more abstract design. By removing the serving recommendations, the USDA intended that consumers decrease their grain and starch consumption, without explaining to them the reasons why 6-11 servings of refined grains, starches and sugar are detrimental to human health.

In June 2011, the USDA published MyPlate, a diagram of a plate and cup divided into five food groups: fruits, grains, vegetables, protein and dairy. The guide is displayed mainly on packaged food items and is currently taught throughout the United States. Unfortunately, there is no mention of healthy oils or dietary fats of any kind to ensure sufficient intake of essential fatty acids, which are required for strengthening cellular membranes of all cells in the body and many other fundamental metabolic processes.

Is this diet, proposed by a government agency, *the* diet to restore health in America? Will the USDA update this nutritional guideline again in the future? If they do, what will it look like and why will they not release the healthiest nutritional guideline once and for all? Can we trust the USDA for proper nutritional guidelines to instruct us on which foods to eat?

In order to discover what the best nutritional guideline is, we must find the healthiest people and study the foods they eat. Instead of looking at individuals, we must look for societies or populations with absolutely perfect health — zero incidence of cardiovascular disease, diabetes or cancer. They must have strong men, women and children, not a single case of infertility, no need for orthodontics and never a tooth cavity. We must study populations completely free of every known chronic illness and degenerative disease.

Do such societies exist?

Absolutely.

Dr. Weston A. Price was the first to locate them and study how they lived and the foods they ate.

MALNUTRITION AND DISEASE

Dr. Weston A. Price practiced dentistry in Cleveland, Ohio during the 1920s. He taught thousands of students at dental schools and authored technical papers and textbooks. His greatest contribution to society stemmed from his curiosity to understand why his patients developed dental cavities and their possible connection to chronic disease. He observed that his patients suffered increasingly more chronic and degenerative diseases over the duration of his practice. Younger patients, the children of the people he had been treating years earlier, had increasingly deformed dental arches, crooked teeth and cavities. The children were also exhibiting poorer health and a greater disposition to illness than their parents. He wanted to know what the cause could be.

Dr. Price sold his practice and traveled around the world with his wife to remote locations to find native cultures, so-called primitive people, who lived happily and free of disease. They specifically looked for healthy people who had not yet been adulterated by modern civilization and technologies. They traveled to visit fourteen groups of native peoples from isolated villages in the Swiss Alps to the Andes

Mountains in Peru, the forests of northern Canada, the Polynesian islands, the Arctic Circle, Scotland, Australia, New Zealand, Alaska and several locations in Africa.

Upon reaching a new group, Dr. Price first gained the trust of the elders. Then, he counted cavities and physically examined the members of their societies. He found less than 1% of tooth decay in all the people he visited. Their teeth were perfectly straight and white, with well-formed facial features and high dental arches. Not one of them required orthodontic or dental braces to achieve perfectly straight teeth. Additionally, none of them practiced any sort of dental hygiene. Not one of his subjects had ever used a toothbrush.

Dr. Price also noticed that, in addition to healthy teeth and gums, all the people were solidly strong, well built and absolutely free of any chronic illness. Dr. Price found no incidence of degenerative diseases, including heart disease, stroke, cancer, diabetes, hemorrhoids, multiple sclerosis, Parkinson's, Alzheimer's, hypothyroidism, fibromyalgia, osteoporosis or chronic fatigue syndrome (called neurasthenia in his day).

Their only health problems were minor ills like headaches, colds, wounds, burns and other minor trauma for which they had developed native remedies from plants and foods found locally according to their climate.

Dr. Price observed in great detail what these people ate and found that each group of people had diets distinct from the other. The Swiss mountain villagers subsisted primarily on unpasteurized and cultured dairy products, especially butter, cheese, whey and yogurt. Rye was an integral part of their diet. They occasionally ate beef from their aging cows. Bone broths, vegetables and berries were commonly consumed. Due to the high altitude, they ate what few vegetables they could grow in the short summer months, fermenting any surplus for winter consumption. The main foods, however, were cheese, butter and rye bread.

Gaelic folks of the Outer Hebrides ate no dairy products, but primarily codfish and other seafood, especially shellfish. Due to low soil fertility, their only grain was oat but it was a major part of the diet. An important dish for growing children and expectant mothers was the head of a cod stuffed with oats and mashed fish liver. Fruits and vegetables grew sparsely.

The Inuit (Eskimo) ate a diet of almost 100% animal products with hefty amounts of fish, walrus, seal and other marine mammals, usually fermented. The blubber (fat) was consumed with homemade relish. They buried their meat and allowed it to slightly putrefy, creating a very nutritious "high meat." They consumed some portions of sea animals raw. (The word "eskimo" translates as "to eat it raw.") The Inuit gathered nuts, berries and some grasses during the short summer months, but those represented a small portion of their diet. They also ate partially digested grasses by cutting open caribou stomachs and intestines, which provided beneficial probiotic bacteria and pre-manufactured Vitamin K and other nutrients.

The Maori of New Zealand, along with other south sea islanders, consumed all sorts of seafood including fish, shark, octopus, sea worms and shellfish. They also consumed fatty pork and a wide variety of vegetables and fruits, including entire coconuts.

African cattle-keeping tribes like the Masai consumed mainly beef, raw milk, organ meats, blood (mainly during times of drought) and virtually no plant foods at all. The Dinkas of the Sudan, whom Dr. Price claimed were the healthiest of all the African tribes he studied, ate a combination of fermented whole grains with fish, along with smaller amounts of red meat, vegetables and fruit. The Bantu tribe (the least hardy of the African tribes studied, yet with no cases of disease or chronic illness) were primarily agriculturists eating mostly beans, squash, corn, millet, vegetables and fruits, with small amounts of milk and meat.

All of these peoples except the Inuit consumed insects — ants, ant eggs, bees, wasps, dragonflies, beetles, crickets, cicadas, moths, termites — and their larvae, especially in more tropical areas. They found that consuming wood eating insects, referred to as grubs, could restore the vitality of platelets and the blood.

All cultures consumed fermented foods each day such as cheese and cultured butter from raw milk, yogurt, kefir, fermented grain drinks like kefir beer made from millet or fermented fish.

The last major feature of native diets was that they were rich in fat, especially animal fat. These included butter, cream, lard and tallow, as well as organ meats supplied by insects, eggs, fish, game animals or domesticated herds. These primitive people knew that they would become sick if they did not consume enough fat, which we now know contain fat-soluble nutrients including vitamins A, E, D, K, F and many more.

These native diets were rich in living enzymes from fermented and raw foods (animal and plant). Enzymes assist in the digestion of food and the body's thousands of metabolic processes. Cooked foods lack these enzymes and force our bodies to deplete their reserves. The traditional foods that the natives consumed contained high food enzyme content from raw dairy, raw meat and fish, raw honey, raw fruits, cold-pressed oils, fermented and unpasteurized wines and beers, plus vegetables, fruits, beverages, dairy, meats and condiments naturally preserved by fermentation. Many diets included seeds, grains and nuts that were soaked, sprouted, germinated, fermented or naturally leavened to neutralize anti-nutrients (enzyme inhibitors, tannins, phytic acid, etc.)

While all cultures consumed vegetables, Dr. Price never found a totally vegetarian society that was free of disease and chronic illness. Notably, the foods of traditional diets were natural and unprocessed. Their foods contain no preservatives, additives or artificial colorings nor processed sweeteners such as sugar, cane sugar or high fructose corn syrup. They contained neither white flour, canned foods nor refined, dehydrogenated or hydrogenated vegetables oils. Their milk products were not pasteurized, homogenized or low fat. The animal and plant foods were nourished on pesticide-free soil and no growth hormones or antibiotics were used. They did not consume any genetically modified organisms or genetically engineered foods, nor were fungicides, herbicides or pesticides sprayed onto their foods. In short, these people always ate organic.

All of Dr. Price's findings and photos are compiled in his masterly documented *Nutrition and Physical Degeneration*. Once he discovered the foods the native people ate for health, he focused on documenting the effects, if any, of converting from a traditional diet to a diet with processed and refined foods. He discovered that physical degeneration is inevitable.

His photographs capture increased rates of tooth decay. Even more startling, they show the change in facial development that occurred with modernization. Parents who began to consume less of the traditional foods gave birth to children with narrower faces, crowded teeth and pinched nostrils. The photographs from his work clearly demonstrate that the foods of modern commerce do not provide sufficient nutrients to allow the body to reach its full genetic potential. He found that insufficient nutrition prevented the complete growth and development of bones in the body and the head as well as the fullest expressions of the immune, nervous, digestive and reproductive systems, which allow humankind to function at optimal levels. Dr. Price's work confirmed that the root cause of any physical malformation, degeneration, illness or disease is directly a result of malnutrition. All modern diseases are different manifestations of specific traditional whole foods missing from a person's diet. To connect with others who have studied the work of Dr. Price in your area, visit www.westonaprice.org.

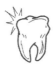

CAVITIES ARE SYMPTOMS

To many modern day Americans, a dental cavity represents an extreme nuisance — a reason to visit our dreaded dentist who will remind us to floss every day, brush our teeth for five minutes longer and choose sugarless gum, despite the fact that most sugarless gum contains aspartame, a very potent ant poison. [125, 126] Bottom line: a dental cavity is a symptom of poor nutrition. Symptoms are important because they are the body's excellent signals that it is not receiving sufficient nutritional value from previous and current food sources.

The dashboard of our modern day automobiles have a check engine light to indicate when there's a problem. When it suddenly illuminates, do you simply turn off the light, ignore inspecting the engine and hope to continue driving without a problem ever developing? Typically, when the light turns on, we hire a mechanic to resolve any underlying issue in order to avoid engine failure. Not resolving the root cause could end up quite costly to fix or lead to irreparable damage.

Filling a cavity is merely turning off the check engine light. This suppression of the symptom allows other health issues to develop. Dr. Price found that while the fillings help prevent excruciating pain, it does not prevent new cavities from forming, which is why he explored the deeper causes of tooth decay.

Holistic health care practitioners understand the value of whole food nutrition in supporting the healing body's ability to regenerate. They assess the health of every organ and work with their patients to restore the organs to optimal performance. True physical mechanics, holistic health care practitioners, identify the source of problems under the hoods of our bodies.

Question #1 to ask your holistic health care practitioner:
Have you studied the work and findings of Dr. Weston Price which attribute the cause of all cavities, disease and degeneration to malnutrition?

DRUG-INDUCED NUTRIENT DEPLETION

Dr. Price discerned that all modern disease is a result of malnutrition. Decades after his book, scientists began to document the specific nutritional deficiencies and thus diseases caused by pharmaceutical drugs. *Drug-Induced Nutrient Depletion Handbook*, compiled by four pharmacists, contains references to clinical studies demonstrating all the known nutrients to be depleted by commonly prescribed pharmaceuticals. It points to how pharmaceutical agents work in opposition to the natural healing process and offers an explanation of how they cause drug-induced diseases. See Figure 12.

The authors state their limitations thus: "We actually believe that the problem of drug-induced nutrient depletions is substantially larger and more widespread than what is reported in this book. Our reason for saying this is that in many cases a drug's effect on various nutrients has not yet been studied."[127] Additionally, the Handbook lacks data on the untold nutrients still yet to be discovered in whole foods, which means potentially hundreds, if not thousands, more nutrients may be depleted.

Drug	Known Nutrient Deficiencies
Antacids	Calcium, Iron, Magnesium, amino acids
Antibiotics	"Friendly/beneficial" bacteria, Vitamin K, minerals
Antidepressants	Vitamin B2, CoEnzyme Q10, Melatonin
Antidiabetic drugs	Vitamin B12, Folic Acid, CoQ10
Anti-inflammatories	Vitamin C, Folic Acid, Iron, Magnesium, Selenium
Analgesic	Folic Acid, Vitamin C, Iron, Potassium
Anti-hypertensives	CoQ10, Magnesium, Vitamin B6
Cholesterol-Lowering Drugs	CoQ10, Vitamin A, Vitamin D, Vitamin E, Vitamin K, Zinc
Diuretics	Vitamin B1, Vitamin B6, Magnesium, Potassium
Female Hormones	Vitamin B6, Vitamin B12, CoQ10, Zinc, Folic Acid
Oral Contraceptives	Vitamin B2, Vitamin B6, Vitamin B12, Magnesium
Laxatives	Potassium
Tranquilizers	Vitamin B2, CoQ10
Anti-convulsants	Folic Acid, Vitamin D, Vitamin K, Calcium, Biotin
Bronchodilators	Vitamin B6, Vitamin B12, CoQ10, Zinc, Folic Acid
Thyroid Hormones	Calcium

Source: Drug-Induced Nutrient Depletion Handbook, 2nd Edition, by R. Pelton

Figure 12. Common pharmaceuticals and related nutrient deficiencies.

Food for Thought: Albert Einstein said, "We cannot solve our problems with the same thinking we used when we created them." It is impossible for a pharmaceutical drug to address symptoms caused by a nutritional deficiency. If a pharmaceutical drug creates a nutritional deficiency, it is impossible to resolve this new problem with another pharmaceutical. Only whole and nutrient dense foods will resolve the problem in both instances.

10

PIONEERING NUTRITION

"There is only one major disease and that is malnutrition."

— D. W. Cavanaugh, M.D. of Cornell University

Weston A. Price returned to the United States and taught his findings nationwide. His book was a required text in Harvard's anthropology department for many years, but has been forgotten in the modern rush for 'progress' in the medical and nutrition realms. Among the doctors who were interested in understanding the application of food as medicine was DeForest Clinton (D.C.) Jarvis, a holistic medical doctor from Vermont whose book *Folk Medicine* popularized the use of raw honey and apple cider vinegar to support healing, even for diabetes, weight loss and insulin resistance.[128]

Dr. Jarvis and Dr. Price formed the "Jarvis Study Group" which met monthly to discuss nutritional discoveries and patient successes. It proposed measures to ensure all Americans had access to proper nutritional information, focusing on foods that would allow everyone to be optimally healthy and free of disease. These fireside chats gathered many amazing minds, including **Francis Pottenger, Melvin**

Page and **Royal Lee** — the pioneers in the field of whole food nutrition.

THE CATS OF POTTENGER

Dr. Francis M. Pottenger, Jr. was a holistic medical doctor who wanted to test the potency of his adrenal hormone extract on donated laboratory cats. Most of the cats died during or following the operation to remove their adrenal glands. He fed the cats a diet consisting of cooked meat scraps of liver, tripe, sweetbread (thymus and other glands), brains, heart and muscle.

When the number of donated cats exceeded the supply of food available, Dr. Pottenger fed raw meat scraps from a local meat packing plant, including organs, meat and bone. Within months, this separate group appeared in better health, their kittens were more energetic and, most interestingly, their post-operative death rate was lower.

To study what foods strengthened or weakened the animals, he began a controlled study involving approximately 900 cats over a period of ten years, which included more than three generations.

In his "Meat Study," one group of cats was fed raw meat, raw (unpasteurized) milk and cod liver oil, while the second group was fed cooked meat, raw milk and cod-liver oil. While the cats fed the all-raw diet were healthy, those fed the cooked diet developed various health problems.

- By the end of the first generation, they started to develop degenerative diseases and became lethargic.
- By the end of the second generation, they had developed degenerative diseases by mid-life and began losing coordination.
- By the end of the third generation, they developed degenerative diseases very early in life and had a much shorter life span. Some were even born blind and weak and others were infertile or incapable of producing offspring. They had an abundance of parasites and vermin, while skin diseases and allergies increased from 5% in healthy cats to over 90% in the malnourished cats.

Kittens of the third generation did not survive beyond six months. Bones became soft and pliable and males became docile while females became more aggressive.

- The cats suffered from most of the degenerative diseases encountered in humans and completely died out by the fourth generation.

At the time of Dr. Pottenger's clinical study, the amino acid taurine was a known essential amino acid for cats. The cooking of meat destroys taurine and other heat sensitive nutrients, preventing cats from properly forming protein structures, resulting in the observed ill-health effects. Humans also require heat sensitive amino acids and other nutrients that are potentially lost during the heating and cooking processes.

In his "Milk Study," all groups were fed raw meat plus one type of milk: raw, pasteurized, evaporated, sweetened condensed or metabolized vitamin D milk. '' The cats on raw milk were the healthiest, while the rest exhibited varying degrees of health problems similar to the cooked meat study. [129]

The work that Dr. Pottenger conducted on the health benefits of raw meat and raw milk for cats demonstrate the long-term risks which heating, cooking and processing of food can have on health. Dr. Pottenger's findings add insight to the findings of Dr. Price, especially his observation of raw milk, meat and organ tissue consumption by native people.

REVERSING INFERTILITY

Unfortunately, today's average American diet is high in cooked (or processed) meats and pasteurized milk. While there is no conclusive data demonstrating whether infertility in humans is directly

''Metabolized vitamin D milk is produced by feeding irradiated yeast to cows.

correlated to the consumption of cooked meat and pasteurized dairy products, it cannot be denied that the incidence of infertility is skyrocketing. As many as 6.7 million (nearly 11% of) American women are experiencing difficulties getting pregnant.[130] Even more are experiencing menstrual cycle abnormalities while male sperm counts are declining.

In his last study, Dr. Pottenger fed raw meat, raw milk and cod liver oil to cats who had developed infertility due to malnutrition. He found that their fertility could be restored within the first generation. However, it took four generations of kittens fed the same raw foods to reach the state of optimal health and vibrancy of his original test subjects.

Weston Price found that when a native individual abandoned ancestral eating habits in favor of modern foods, ill health and dental cavities followed. If that same person resumed their original eating pattern, health returned and the progression of dental decay stopped and reversed. This is perhaps the most uplifting aspect of both Dr. Pottenger's and Dr. Price's work — we can reverse the negative trend through diet. The foods we choose to eat today may impact the health of four generations of our progeny, for better or worse.

NUTRITIONAL BIOCHEMISTRY

In our polluted modern world, there are additional factors that contribute to infertility, disease and degeneration. These include radiation, alcohol, smoking, drugs, pharmaceuticals, pesticides, heavy metals, chemotherapy, etc. [131] Environmental exposure is often unavoidable and affects our internal biochemistry. One member of the Jarvis Study Group, Dr. Melvin E. Page, DDS, found that specific foods were capable of restoring the body's ability to deal with additional environmental stressors and provide balanced nutritional biochemistry.

In 1919, Dr. Page began a successful dental practice in Muskegon, Michigan. He became known as one of the top orthodontists, especially for his invention of dentures. However, he found himself making a new set of dentures every two and a half years for many of his patients as their jaw bones continued to diminish.

In a quest to learn why oral diseases progressively deteriorate, Dr. Page met with Dr. Price and studied his work on native people. At local hospitals in Michigan, he ran more than two thousand blood chemistries and discovered that no deterioration of bone occurred (and no cavities formed) when the ratio in the blood of calcium to phosphorus was 10 to 4. The Department of Dental Research of the United States Air Force confirmed his findings 42 years later. Dr. Page also found blood sugar levels should be at 85 mg/dL, plus or minus 5 mg/dL. By restoring ideal calcium/phosphorus ratio and blood sugar levels, the deterioration of bone stops.

Dr. Page discovered that processed foods, refined carbohydrates and white sugar increase serum calcium by drawing the mineral from bone tissue. The idea that diet and nutrition could cause a biochemical condition affecting the teeth, and that he dared to suggest his patients should change their eating habits were not widely accepted in modern medicine, which focuses on treating symptoms and avoids addressing causes. For this his professional colleagues ostracized him, but he continued his research into how the body's biochemistry, when balanced through proper nutrition, will not only prevent dental problems but also naturally affect overall health.

Though he did not offer the convenient quick fix sought by so many individuals, his treatment and philosophy were simple and logical. He believed that fad diets, overnight cures and radical therapies do nothing but create harmful side effects. In his practice, he helped thousands of patients by following a few key principles:

- Avoid processed foods, refined carbohydrates and white sugar.
- Avoid foods with chemical additives for the sake of "shelf life" because they disrupt the body's biochemistry.
- Supplement food intake with whole food-based concentrates, minerals and digestive enzymes as necessary.
- Milk is not the perfect food for everyone. Pasteurized milk should be avoided by all.

- Balance the endocrine system without the use of synthetic (or "bioidentical") hormones for optimum physical and mental health.

- Follow the Food Plan.

The Page Food Plan, developed on the glycemic index, encourages patients to eat unlimited quantities of green leafy vegetables.

In the early 1960s Dr. Page was indicted by the federal government for practicing outside the scope of practice for conventional dentistry. After a lengthy trial, in which he introduced over 3,600 case studies and was able to substantiate his findings with over 40,000 blood tests as well as 35 years of research, a federal judge found him not guilty. The judge went on to reprimand the American Medical Association and the FDA for harassing him rather than trying to figure out what he was doing. He went ahead with his ideas despite tremendous adversity launched by colleagues in the dental and medical profession, as well as the press and others who mocked his forward-thinking ideas. Using the system he developed, he was consistently successful in healing many of the degenerative diseases most common today.

Only today are we gaining a fuller understanding of the value of Dr. Page's research into calcium-phosphorus levels. His unique system of graphing the endocrine system has proven extremely valuable in understanding a person's genetic potential for life.

In 1968, he questioned the allopathic medical world, "Why does modern medicine find it so hard to look at, and accept, many of these simple truths?" It remains a question that many medical doctors continue to avoid answering to this very day.

Figure 13 is a Phase II diet adapted from Dr. Melvin Page, which I use in my nutritional practice to guide clients on the vegetables they should begin to consume immediately to rebalance their body's biochemistry.

Question #2 to ask your holistic health care practitioner:
Are you familiar with Dr. Page's Food Plan and how to restore proper mineral ratios for a healthy body?

PHASE II Diet for Balancing Blood Chemistry

Phase II diet for balancing blood chemistry (edited from Melvin Page's work)
Removing Starches will control your blood sugar, which will
remove THE major stress on your body-hypoglycemia
1. Most important step is to remove starches and all pasta, bread, white potatoes and rice
2. Consume protein three times a day
3. Dilute all juice 50% with water. Fruit juices should be hand squeezed
4. Do not drink too much fluid with meals for it reduces digestive capacity

Complete Protein 3x/day	UNLIMITED AMOUNTS		
BEEF (100% grass finished)	**VEGETABLES**	**VEGETABLES**	**FATS & OILS**
BISON (100% grass finished)	**3% or less carbs**	**3% or less carbs**	Raw Butter, Ghee
FISH (wild caught)	Asparagus	Radishes	Coconut Oil
FOWL (free range)	Bamboo Shoots	Raw Cob Corn	Olive Oil (cold pressed)
EGGS (free range)	Bean Sprouts	Arugula	Avocado Tallow, Lard, Duck Fat
Whey Protein (undenatured)	Beet Greens	Sauerkraut	**Beverages**
Animal protein requirements are calculated by taking your weight in pounds and divide by 15 to get min. ounces per day. ie. 150lbs/15=10oz per day; 10oz/3 meals = 3.3 oz per meal	Bok Choy Greens	Spinach	Spring Water Filtered Water
	Broccoli	Yellow Squash	Teas (organic)
	Cabbages	Zucchini Squash	Probiotic Sodas Beet Kvass
	Cauliflower	**6% or less carbs**	Broths (chicken, beef)
VEGETABLES (organic)	Celery	Bell Peppers	**2-3 times per wk max**
(see guidelines to right)	Chards	Bok Choy Stems	**VEGETABLES**
FRUIT (organic)	Chicory	Chives	**7- 9% carbs**
Unlimited amount of ANY fruit as long as double the amount of Vegetables (3% or less) are consumed. Best (low glycemic) snack fruits are: Apple, Goji/Berries/Cherries, Grapes, Peach, Pear, Plum	Collard Greens	Eggplant	Acorn Squash
	Cucumber	Green Beans	Artichokes
	Endive	Green Onions	Beets
	Escarole	Okra	Butternut Squash
	Garlic	Olives	Carrots
	Kale	Pickles	Jicama
	Kohlrabi	Pimento	Leeks
NUTS & SEEDS	Lettuces	Rhubarb	Onion
Between meals snack.	Mushrooms	Sweet Potatoes	Pumpkin
(raw, organic, sprouted)	Mustard Greens	Tomatoes	Rutabagas
Almonds, Hazel, Walnut, Brazil	Parsley	Water Chestnuts	Turnips
Sunflower, Sesame	Sea Vegetables	Yams	Winter Squashes
Hemp, Chia seeds	Dandelion Greens	Brussels Sprouts	Parsnips

Figure 13. Modified Page Food Plan

RAW, WHOLE FOOD-BASED CONCENTRATES

Dr. Page recommended that all his patients supplement their diet with "whole food-based concentrates," referring to the whole food concentrates of Dr. Royal Lee, DDS. Dr. Lee, one of Dr. Page's closest friends and colleagues, was a researcher, inventor, scientist, scholar, statesman, businessman and philanthropist.

From age twelve, in 1907, Dr. Lee compiled a notebook on biochemistry and nutrition that became one of the largest individual collections in the world.

In 1924, before Weston Price had returned with his findings, Dr. Lee presented a paper on "The Systemic Causes of Dental Caries," in which he outlined the relationship of vitamin deficiencies to tooth decay and showed the necessity of vitamins from food sources for normal functioning of the endocrine glands.

Dr. Lee, a prolific inventor, patented a speed controller for dentist drills. With an inclination toward philanthropy, he developed something to help fellow Americans correct their nutritional deficiencies, for he knew government agencies and for-profit food manufacturers were only concerned with extending shelf life rather than preserving nutrient density and vitality of the food they processed. Dr. Lee believed that a healthy life is the result of vitamins, and their functions are far too complex to be reproduced by human beings. So at the age of 21, he began formulating a whole food-based concentrate that would optimize health by delivering all known vitamins and minerals in their natural, bioactive state. Using whole food sources, he knew that undiscovered nutrients would also be present.

At the time he created the formula, no equipment could concentrate these foods without disrupting their nutritional integrity. He and his company Lee Engineering invented the required technology to preserve and not disturb the delicate nutrient complexes in the foods of his formula. Within a few years he had built devices to extract and concentrate food without heat or mechanical refining so that all the enzymes and heat sensitive nutrients remain active. In 1929, this resulted in the world's first ever raw, whole-food concentrate, Catalyn™; although the words "raw" and "whole-food" did not enter the public media until the 21st century.

Dr. Lee knew which foods have the highest amounts of the essential vitamins and minerals from his own research and that of Drs. Price, Page and Jarvis. The vegetables included were based on Dr. Page's Food Plan. Dr. Lee put the traditional foods of the native people studied by Dr. Price into his whole food-based concentrate formulas. The Peruvian mountain people traveled for a month down to the ocean to collect kelp. Dr. Price asked, "Why do you travel so far for that seaweed?" They explained that it helps the heart and all muscles. Dr. Lee understood the value of this and all the observations Dr. Price recorded, so he concentrated kelp into specific mineral products for optimal heart and muscle function.

That year his mother contracted a strange flu. She was diagnosed with a failing heart and given six months to live. Dr. Lee immediately began to feed her Catalyn™ and her health began to improve quickly. She lived another twelve years (into her 80s). Catalyn™ produced remarkable results. Many people with declining health experienced a complete reversal of problems that had been deemed beyond help by medical doctors. Dr. Lee's great love for his family, as well as his love for humanity in general, motivated him to create other whole food-based concentrates. It eventually led to the founding of Standard Process, Inc.

Dr. Lee produced other specialized formulas to address specific causes of nutritional deficiency for dentists, chiropractors, acupuncturists and holistic medical doctors to restore health to their patients. Working closely with them, Dr. Lee documented thousands of case studies affirming the seemingly miraculous results of his products. Today, Standard Process Inc. carries a line of over 150 raw, whole food-based formulas.

FROM SEED TO CONCENTRATE

Conversation with Peter, a nutritional client:

"I eat a pretty healthy diet."

"What exactly does that mean?" I asked.

"Well, what I mean is that I eat out once in awhile and I only have fast food a few times a week and I only drink diet sodas."

"And did you know that eating devitalized processed foods can lead to organ dysfunction, resulting in symptoms and maybe even cavities?"

"No, I didn't." He admitted.

"Do you know where your food comes from?"

He paused. "Costco."

Most of us are not aware about the origin of our food, which may travel long distances — coconuts from Thailand, oranges from Florida, apples from Washington. They are left on grocery store shelves for us to purchase. Then these perishable foods sit on our counters for a few days before they are consumed. We don't know if these foods were genetically modified or artificially selected through crop manipulation. We are uncertain which pesticides, fungicides, herbicides or other chemicals were sprayed on them or if chemical fertilizers were ever mixed into the soils they grew from. We do not know if these foods were exposed to other chemical toxins during transport or if retailers injected artificial coloring to enhance curb appeal to our uninformed eyes.

Is every ingredient in the dish you recently ordered at a restaurant grown, handled and prepared to ensure it contains sufficient nutrient value for your body? Were harmful chemicals used during any step of the way? When restaurant employees apply bleach or other chemical detergents to kitchen equipment, surfaces and floors, are traces of those chemicals entering the food that is prepared? If so, what do our bodies do to prevent those chemicals from developing into a chronic health issue?

When Steve Jobs was CEO of Apple, he kept a tight ship and every employee understood the need for a strict company culture to keep all proprietary information contained. Why? Jobs and Apple prevent other competitors from copying any proprietary technologies, which allows Apple to have a foothold on the market by developing innovative products that no consumer can ever expect. However, Apple designs products that consumers "want" in their lives. If a product is something we "want" (versus need), we can choose to purchase it or not. Despite the fact that some of us may panic when we misplace our iPhone, we are quite capable of surviving without the use of an Apple branded device.

The same cannot be said about food. We must be fully aware of every substance that enters our body, because it is either a nutritious food that rebuilds the body or it is a devitalized food, possibly filled with toxins, that destroys the body. When a farmer produces a food and fails to provide absolute transparency regarding the processes of growing and harvesting, is it actually safe for human consumption?

In the early 1930s, Dr. Lee purchased over 300 acres of organic farmland in the fertile glacier-created lands of Wisconsin where he had grown up. Since then, organic farmers have grown acres of alfalfa, barley grass, beets, Brussels sprouts, buckwheat, kale, Spanish black radish, kidney beans, oats and pea vines on that land for Dr. Lee's whole food-based concentrates. Every organic vegetable is inspected thoroughly with the most advanced laboratory tools.

The company collects their own seeds from organic and heirloom vegetables; rainwater from above and an aquifer below irrigate the soil. Though "organic" certification represents a formal recognition of production quality, Dr. Lee has always ensured his farmers operated the land organically and in accordance with the principles of permaculture and biodynamic farming in order to ensure the highest vitality and nutrient rich vegetables.

To produce the healthiest vegetables, he required the healthiest seeds, an abundance of microorganisms in the compost and topsoil, sufficient flow of pure ground water and long hours of sunlight. We should all know our farmers and support those who produce toxin-free, nutrient dense food to effectively nourish our healing bodies.

If you visit the Lee farm in Palmyra, Wisconsin, you will meet the farmers, learn about their organic composting system, see a map of crop rotation and learn how they harvest the vegetables in the morning when nutrient density is highest. After the harvest, they are taken to a juicer where the fiber is removed and added to the organic compost. The vat of nutrient rich juice is transferred without delay to a vacuum, which removes all water from the mixture to concentrate nutrients into a powder. By removing the water, the nutrients remain in a state of dormancy and are reactivated upon consumption. The food powder is compressed into tablets or mixed into capsules with other nutrient dense foods. They are then packaged in dry, dark colored glass bottles to ensure nutrients are not destroyed by extreme heat, light and dampness.

Where does your food come from? Do your research. If it's Costco, look at all labels and contact the growers to see if you can inspect their growing operations to ensure they are not adding any unsafe chemicals. Unfortunately, many grocery chains now carry frozen vegetables labeled "organic" from China. How can you know whether the vegetables are truly raised organically? Only by knowing your farmer personally.

Take a trip to Wisconsin, visit the farmers, inspect their seeds, grab a handful of the farm's organism-rich soil and you'll truly know what it means to eat organically. If you cannot visit Wisconsin, look for your nearest farmer's market. Every week, you can find many local organic growers who sell fresh harvests of vegetables and fruits. At these local markets, the farmers are happy to build a long lasting relationship with you and willingly talk about their organic farming methods. Many of their vegetables and fruits are handpicked the same morning, which ensures their nutritive value because they were allowed to ripen fully on the vine or tree.

Question #3 to ask your holistic health care practitioner:
Where is your favorite farmer's market?

FRESH INGREDIENTS

During my sophomore year at U.C. Berkeley, I worked as a waiter in a sushi restaurant. I was instructed to become familiar with all of the restaurant's offerings. Within three weeks, I had memorized all the dishes and could handle customer questions with confidence. But one Friday evening, a customer asked, "How fresh is the fish?"

I did not know how to answer, so I politely excused myself and asked the head chef.

"Very fresh!" he yelled out.

I returned to the customer's table and informed him that the fish was "Very fresh!" I'm not sure he knew what that meant but he was satisfied.

The following day, I arrived earlier than normal and was shocked to find a new shipment of fish lying on the kitchen floor, frozen. "Really? Frozen fish is considered fresh?" After the fish thawed out, my manager conducted the most sophisticated test I have ever seen to ensure the fish was safe for human consumption. He put his face next to the fish and took a sniff — the same method I used during college to determine whether a shirt could be worn in public for one more day or be put in the wash due to a traceable odor.

As consumers, we are not aware of the origin of the fish we order in a restaurant. We do not know if it swam in waters polluted with radioactive iodine isotopes from Fukushima, was injected with hormones, fed antibiotics, exposed to environmental toxins during transport or how long it has been dead or frozen. So much is unknown about the foods in restaurants.

Every raw, whole food-based concentrate produced by Dr. Lee has been tested to be safer than anything you purchase at supermarkets or restaurants. At his farm, Dr. Lee instituted an advanced system of inspecting all ingredients for heavy metals, pathogens, chemicals and other harmful substances. Every ingredient is subjected to six to fifteen tests to ensure the foods contained in Dr. Lee's formulas are safer than the fish you eat at your favorite local restaurant. In fact, they blow the sniff test out of the water.

THE WISDOM OF APPLICATION

My grandmother was a calm and confident woman of Portuguese descent who was born and grew up in Shanghai. She witnessed many atrocities, including the second Japanese invasion of Shanghai and turmoil in China from the 1930s to 1945. After

Japanese occupation of China ended, her family attempted to restore a normal life. Soon however, civil war eventually split the country into two, leading to the Communist regime in mainland China. In 1949, she and her family fled as the Communists embarked on a purge of all foreigners, deemed invaders. She settled in Brazil and then moved to the United States.

Right before I graduated high school, my grandmother and I sat down in the family room of her house in San Francisco and she began speaking about events in her life including how she survived two wars. She explained to me that there are things in life we can change and there are those that we cannot. "For the things we cannot change; we must accept them as they are and not dwell. For those that can be changed, we must have the courage to do what is right. We must be wise enough to know the difference between the two."

The survival of her family depended on their ability to change life's obstacles into gateways of opportunity. When she was young, her mother died, so her older sister raised her and six younger siblings, since there was no orphanage to retreat to. Wisdom came quickly or they would have perished. My grandmother learned to speak Japanese, Shanghainese, Mandarin, Portuguese and English.

She asked me if I knew the difference between knowledge and wisdom. I shook my head. She said we spend our entire lives learning to understand the difference between them. Whatever we learn in school or read in books is knowledge. The application of that knowledge to improve human life is wisdom. "Many people of our time and in our world represent wisdom in its highest good. They synthesize, apply knowledge and implement it out of the passion to help others. Do what you can to recognize who they are. More importantly, strive to become one of them."

Dr. Lee would be one of the people my grandmother referred to as someone who applied what he learned for the benefit of fellow humankind.

The research and resulting discoveries of the nutrition pioneers brought forth a new truth that food is *real* medicine for the healing body. This group of stellar minds and humble hearts left us a message: the true cause of all disease and physical degeneration is malnutrition.

Even more crucial is that the solution resides in the food our hunter-gatherer ancestors ate. A tangible possibility for healing and overcoming disease exists in those who apply what they learn. We are all wise. We all can heal.

More information on the research, philosophy and teachings of Dr. Royal Lee can be found at www.seleneriverpress.com, www.drroyallee.com and www.ifnh.org.

11

PHONY FOODS FOR FAKE BODIES

*"The food you eat can be either the safest and most powerful
form of medicine or the slowest form of poison."*

— Ann Wigmore

"You are what you eat." Have you ever considered the meaning of these commonly spoken words? They serve as a simple message to remind us if we consume foods that have been provided by nature in its unrefined form, we will grow to be strong and healthy. Conversely, if we consume foods that are highly processed, refined, denatured and adulterated, we should expect the opposite.

The most memorable movie dialogue of my childhood occurs in the movie, *Superman II* (1980), right after Clark Kent enters a diner. A customer sitting at the counter, named Rocky, yells to the waitress, "Gimme another plate of this garbage!"

Clark responds, "Gee, that's funny. I've never seen garbage eat garbage before." Rocky utters an insult and punches Clark. Clark, who recently regained his powers as Superman, throws Rocky across the room into a pinball machine. All the diner employees and truck driver customers are stunned by his power to quell an obnoxious patron. He calmly hands the owner of the diner a wad of cash and says, "I'm, uh, terribly sorry about all the damage, Sir. Oh, I've been, uh… uh, working out."

As a child, I believed that scene was hilarious because Clark Kent called Rocky, a human being, garbage. He implied Rocky was filthy, putrid and annoyingly disgusting by equating him to a rotting pile of trash. The creative repetition of the word "garbage" rang like a musical echo to my ears. I found myself utterly amused at the potential for a superhero to poetically forewarn an imminent pummeling.

When I grew up I asked: What if people *really* ate garbage? What would happen to us? Would Superman be there to straighten us up, guide us to a healthy lifestyle and teach us how to be strong and free of illness?

Much of our society's manufactured waste, thrown into landfills, is toxic to humans. Who in their right mind would consume a food or substance that contains toxins? Food manufacturers create products that contain many toxins. They aren't lethal, which means they won't kill us immediately. But they contain preservatives, pesticides and other chemical substances that are known to cause cancer and other disease. When we know how commercially made products are bad for us and what the long-term ramifications are, we're motivated to avoid them. Food manufacturers use incomplete nutritional labels and employ various labeling gimmicks. They deceive us into believing that we are garbage pails with hairy lids on top, so that we continue to feed ourselves the rubbish they produce. We must learn to differentiate a nourishing whole food from the processed garbage that masquerades as food products in grocery store aisles.

To throw even more salt on the open wound, manufactured food products have had essential nutrients removed to improve shelf life and sales revenues. I, too, ate edible manufactured garbage for many years, and I have suffered the physical degeneration that develops from malnutrition and chemical toxicity. I used to have an awesome childhood fantasy, which included owning a crystal fortress and possessing great superpowers of flight, x-ray vision and uncanny strength like the man of steel. Many other children have also dreamed to become the successor to their favorite comic book superheroes. However, outside our dreams we must realize that real food is what will grant us strength, power, and ultimately, health. Delectable imitations and phony foods have become our kryptonite. How did these foods enter the standard American diet? How can we avoid them?

THE ILLUSION OF "ENRICHED BREAD"

Nature packages foods to contain dozens and sometimes hundreds of phytonutrients, minerals, enzymes, amino acids, fatty acids, and perhaps other undiscovered nutrients needed to run the biochemical processes inside our cells like the Krebs cycle, electron transport, glycolysis and gluconeogenesis which break down certain nutrients and convert them into energy. Refining and processing destroys or removes the majority of these vital nutrients. As a result, the body's reserves become depleted, leading to physical symptoms.

For example, a whole-wheat kernel containing hundreds of known nutrients, is composed of three parts:

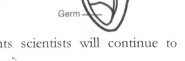

1. Bran (mainly fiber)
2. Endosperm (the starch and gluten)
3. Germ (enzymes, vitamins, minerals and essential fatty acids)

Who knows what other nutrients scientists will continue to discover in whole food sources each year?

Unfortunately, in order to improve the shelf life of wheat flour products, food manufacturers remove and discard the bran and germ, leaving only the starch and gluten. Oftentimes the refined flour is bleached to ensure no enzymes remain alive in the product, thus preventing it from decomposing. This process leaves the flour white. Manufacturers then spray a few synthetically made vitamins back into the refined flour and label it as "enriched" or "fortified".

The word "enriched" means "to improve the quality of; to make a valuable addition to". If someone steals $1,000 from you and returns six monopoly dollars back, do you feel enriched? Do you feel fortified? This is known as nutritional robbery.

The germ of a wheat kernel is an excellent source of the Vitamin B complex, essential fatty acids (linoleic, palmitic, oleic, alpha-linolenic), fat soluble Vitamin E complex, octacosanol, minerals (potassium, iron, calcium, zinc, magnesium, chromium, phosphorous, manganese, copper, selenium) and many more essential nutrients which are used and stored in organs and tissues. The consumption of processed foods robs the body's store of nutrients, leaving organs hungry for more nutrient dense foods. If your organs are never fed these, they begin to break down or fatigue, giving rise to symptoms. Avoid all white flour products, including those that claim to have been enriched or fortified.

TRICKS ARE FOR KIDS

Nutritional labels are often misleading by design. Food manufacturers' nutritional labels include specific product information to influence a consumer's purchasing decision, and ultimately create a long-term craving for the product.

Some labels are designed to increase the number of servings consumed. Trix, a favorite breakfast cereal, is a packaged food I ate on occasion as a child. I enjoyed pouring milk into a large bowl and adding the cereal until my bowl overflowed. As I inhaled the sugary breakfast, I read the back of the box and completed whatever maze the General Mills' marketers had cleverly designed. These silly games usually occupied my attention for a short 30 seconds. Then I proceeded to the side of the box and read the nutritional label. See Figure 14.

The bottom half of the label states that one serving provides 25% of daily value for certain minerals and vitamins. I thought to myself, "I'm a growing boy, and I'm getting bullied by larger classmates, why would I want to consume only 25% of my day's required nutrition? Why not consume 100% or more?" In a mere 30 seconds, I justified the consumption of three additional servings of a highly refined grain and sugar food product. Furthermore, television advertisements by food manufacturers, elementary school nutrition teachers, and cartoon rabbits had trained me and other young children to believe "*Trix are for kids*" without explaining to us the potential long-term risks of cavity formation and other symptoms related to malnutrition.

Many nutritional labels on processed food products are designed so consumers falsely believe they provide adequate nutritional value. No nutritional label exists on real, unprocessed, whole and unadulterated foods. Try to find a freshly picked tomato with a *'trans fat free'* nutritional label. You won't, because the farmers and you both know it hasn't been processed. Only processed foods contain man-made *'trans fats.'*

Many of us purchase fresh meats, vegetables, fruits, eggs and cheese from a local farmer's market or health store because we are concerned with the nutritional content

Nutrition Facts
Serving Size ¾ Cup (30g)

Amount Per Serving	Cereal	with ½ cup skim milk
Calories	110	150
Calories from Fat	0	0

	% Daily Value**	
Total Fat 0g*	0%	0%
Saturated Fat 0g	0%	0%
Trans Fat 0g		
Polyunsaturated Fat 0g		
Monounsaturated Fat 0g		
Cholesterol 0mg	0%	0%
Sodium 140mg	6%	9%
Potassium 35mg	1%	7%
Total Carbohydrate 27g	9%	11%
Dietary Fiber less than 1g	3%	3%
Sugars 11g		
Protein 1g		

Vitamin A	10%	15%
Vitamin C	10%	10%
Calcium	0%	15%
Iron	25%	25%
Vitamin D	10%	25%
Thiamin	25%	30%
Riboflavin	25%	35%
Niacin	25%	25%
Vitamin B₆	25%	25%
Folic Acid	25%	25%
Vitamin B₁₂	25%	35%

* Amount in cereal. One half cup of skim milk contributes an additional 40 calories, 65mg sodium, 6g total carbohydrate (6g sugars), and 4g protein.
** Percent Daily Values are based on a 2,000 calorie diet. Your daily values may be higher or lower depending on your calorie needs:

	Calories	2,000	2,500
Total Fat	Less than	65g	80g
Sat. Fat	Less than	20g	25g
Cholesterol	Less than	300mg	300mg
Sodium	Less than	2,400mg	2,400mg
Potassium		3,500mg	3,500mg
Total Carbohydrate		300g	375g
Dietary Fiber		25g	30g

Ingredients: Milled corn, sugar, contains 2% or less of malt flavoring, salt, BHT for freshness.

Figure 14. Popular commercial cereal nutritional label.

of these foods in their conventional form. How often do you request a nutritional label before buying a head of lettuce or a bunch of bananas? Did you read the nutritional label for the kale, carrots or Brussels sprouts on your recent grocery run? Have you ever seen the nutritional label for a tri-tip steak, salmon filet or chicken breast?

Most of us do not bother to look for the nutritional label when we purchase real and fresh whole food items. We intuitively know what *real* whole food is. Nutritional labels are merely selling tools for corporate food manufacturers to trick us (like kids) into justifying the purchase of processed food.

However, for real food items, we must still investigate the quality of the food to learn if it comes close to the nutritional standard of primitive cultures. For this, we must ask a different set of questions.

1) Were these vegetables organically grown — raised without synthetic fertilizers, pesticides, fungicides, or herbicides?

2) Is the chicken from free-ranged poultry, free to roam during its entire lifetime? Or confined to a cage?

3) Is the beef from a pastured cow, free to graze in leisure and consume grass? Or is it from a factory farm, crammed in with other cows, wading in its own feces and overfed grains to encourage unnaturally rapid weight gain?

4) Is the salmon wild caught from unpolluted waters? Or is it farm-raised or even worse, genetically modified by molecular engineers?

5) Is the milk raw and unpasteurized? Is the milk from a cow that was not injected with hormones, vaccines, antibiotics, or artificially stimulated to unnaturally increase its milk output?

6) Is the cheese, yogurt and kefir made from raw whole milk from pastured cows? Or from pasteurized milk?

Since these questions pertain to the quality of how a food is grown or raised, they can only be answered by the farmers, hunters or gatherer themselves. The local farmers who sell their produce at a farmer's market are great resources to learn about the care and nourishment put into your food that in turn nourishes your body. When reading any label, look to see if the package contains whole food sources. Then, ask how and where the foods were grown or raised. Be wary of all packaged foods. The primitive peoples studied by Dr. Price consumed no packaged foods whatsoever — nothing from cardboard boxes, plastic bags, tin cans or plastic bottles. These primitive peoples had only one food manufacturer in their villages. That was the farmland they tilled. The vegetables they grew and the animals they caught or raised were all provided by their local environment. The only and honest food manufacturer that produces nutrient dense foods rich in minerals, vitamins, essential fatty acids and protein comes straight from the very life-giving ground we walk on.

Food for Thought: On many packaged food labels, information about chemical additives are intentionally left incomplete or entirely missing in order to prevent scaring a consumer away from purchasing a product. At the bottom of the label in Figure 14 it reads, "BHT for freshness." BHT stands for butylated hydroxytoluene, a known carcinogen and tumor growth promoter.[132,133] In this packaged food, and many others sold to children, BHT serves to increase shelf life. If you care about your children, be cautious what you feed them, especially when advertisements claim that they're *"for kids."*

IF A PRODUCT IS FDA APPROVED IN A FOREST, IS IT SAFE AND SOUND?

The FDA is a government agency. Its role is to protect the public from harmful food substances, drugs and other chemicals. It was originally established during the late 1800s to protect the public's health. However, in the early 1900s, it began to protect the commercial food manufacturing industry instead by allowing the production of devitalized processed foods. During this time, our greatest nutrition political advocate was Dr. Harvey Wiley. He was the last general to fight in the war to ensure that pure foods are served at our kitchen tables.

During the late 1800s, he taught chemistry at Harvard and spent his time mastering the use of the polariscope, a device to study sugar chemistry. He identified and documented all the methods by which sugar could be adulterated. While he taught at Purdue University, he was asked by the Indiana State Board of Health to analyze the sugars and syrups for sale throughout the state and to sound an alarm when he detected adulteration.

In 1882, Dr. Wiley was appointed chemist of the U.S. Department of Agriculture (USDA) Division of Chemistry because of his abilities to employ an objective approach in investigating tampering of food. He conducted experiments through 1895 and discovered all sorts of food adulteration with additives. A handful of legislative successes had been won in the early 1890's from his collaboration with the American Society for the Prevention of the Adulteration of Food and other organizations. However, the enforcement of these laws lacked strict implementation. In 1901, the USDA Division of Chemistry became the USDA Bureau of Chemistry, where a food laboratory was created to establish food standards. Dr. Wiley consulted not only with manufacturers but also consumers. He conducted studies on the effects of preservatives on the human body, and his findings on the dangers were very influential. The first results of these experiments were published in 1904. More than a century later, many chemical food preservatives confirmed as carcinogens are still added to various processed food products.

Dr. Wiley was a tireless advocate of national pure food and drug legislation, which he considered his life's work. He was a crusader in supporting national food regulation. With the backing of President Theodore Roosevelt, the landmark Pure Food and Drugs Act was passed by Congress in 1906 and signed into law. The bill prohibited adulteration and misbranding of food and drugs, and was the most comprehensive legislation of its kind in the United States.

After the bill was passed, Dr. Wiley continued his advocacy of the issue, emphasizing the need for strict standards in product labeling. He wrote *Foods and Their Adulteration* in 1907, which explained in clear detail the preparation and adulteration of foods for the general consumer. Under his leadership, the Bureau of Chemistry grew significantly, both in strength and stature.

One episode in Dr. Wiley's crusade involved the seizure of three train containers full of bleached flour. He and other scientists knew that the bleaching process left nitrate residue in the flour. The case *U.S. vs. Lexington Mill and Elevator Company* went all the way to the Supreme Court, which ruled in favor of the government and ordered the flour to be destroyed. However, USDA Secretary, James Wilson ignored the decision and allowed the bleached flour to be made available for consumer purchase. Many suspected a closed-door cash donation was made from the refining grain mills directly into Wilson's back pocket.

Dr. Wiley also filed a case against Coca-Cola™ to prevent the artificial beverage from being sold in multiple states. In his lawsuit, he stated that "No food in our country would have any trace of benzoic acid, sulfurous acid or sulfites or any alum or saccharin, save for medical purposes. No soft drink would contain caffeine or theobromine. No bleached flour would enter interstate commerce. Our foods and drugs would be wholly without any form of adulteration and misbranding. The health of our people would be vastly improved and the life greatly extended. The manufacturers of our food supply, and especially the millers, would devote their energies to improving the public health and promoting happiness in every home by the production of whole ground, unbolted cereals and meals."[134] The term "unbolted" refers to grains that are unrefined and left whole to include the bran and germ with all their essential nutrients required by the human body.

From the beginning of his appointment into office, and through the enforcement of the Pure Food and Drugs Act, he had seen the fundamental principles of that act antagonized, stonewalled or discredited. He was forced to resign from his post on March 15, 1912. The Bureau of Chemistry ceased to exist and in 1931 it re-emerged as the Food and Drug Administration (FDA). From here on out, the power shifted in favor of the commercial manufacturers of devitalized processed foods. Soon it would be against the law to claim that white flour was less nutritious than whole-wheat flour. Government institutions, originally formed to protect the public health and ensure that only safe and healthy foods entered the American food supply, became proponents of refined and chemical filled foodstuffs that inevitably lead to malnutrition, physical degeneration and chronic illness.

After Dr. Wiley resigned from the USDA, he took over the laboratories of *Good Housekeeping* magazine. There, he continued his work for 18 years to serve his fellow citizens by demanding truth in food labeling, and to support the nutrition pioneers D.C. Jarvis, Weston Price, Royal Lee and Melvin Page with his legal and political expertise.

Food for Thought: The chemical 4-Methylimidazole, used in popular cola soft drinks as a caramel coloring agent, is known to cause cancer.[135] In March of 2012, USA Today reported that Coca-Cola Co. and PepsiCo Inc. are changing the way they make the caramel coloring used in their sodas as a result of a California law that mandates a cancer warning label on drinks containing a certain level of carcinogens. It is safer to consume whole foods that have not been artificially colored.

GENETICALLY MODIFIED = FRANKENFOOD

The FDA has evolved to protect the interests of the commercial industry, while leaving the consumer uninformed about the long-term effects of manufactured food products. Since the forced departure of Dr. Harvey Wiley, the FDA's focus has increasingly turned away from protecting the public and toward collaborating in the profiteering efforts of biotech corporations, which have, for decades, employed molecular engineers to insert foreign genes into the DNA of vegetable seedlings. The inserted genes come from mutant species that carry specific bacteria and viruses, which have never existed in the human food supply before.

Any food which has its DNA altered is known as a Genetically Modified Organism (GMO). They are also referred to as genetically modified (GM) or genetically engineered (GE). GMOs are common ingredients in most processed foods. The FDA currently does not require *any* safety evaluations or labeling of GMOs. A company can even introduce a GM food to the market without telling consumers or the FDA. This leaves us all to serve as guinea pigs.

GM foods were made possible by a technology developed in the 1970s whereby genes from one species are spliced into the DNA of other species. Genes produce proteins, which in turn generate characteristics or traits. The dreams that biotechnology corporations promise the public include the possible discovery of traits to allow vegetables to grow in deserts, be fortified with additional nutrients, and yield more productive crops to feed the starving millions all over the world. Unfortunately, after nearly 20 years, none of these have been achieved.

The only two traits that are found in nearly all commercialized GM plants are herbicide tolerance and self-pesticide production. Herbicide tolerant soy, corn, cotton and canola plants are engineered with bacterial genes that allow them to survive otherwise deadly doses of herbicides. This gives farmers flexibility to apply various pesticides onto the growing vegetables and soil without harming the crop. Furthermore, GM seed companies continue to generate a profit because they own the patents to specific GM seeds.

The growing of GM foods creates two indefinite problems. The first is the inability to contain the spraying and travel of pesticides, leaving them to perpetuate long-term ecological disruptions. The second is that we do not know if GM foods are safe to consume long-term. The nutritional make up of these foods have never been measured or compared to heirloom and organic vegetables consumed by the primitive cultures studied by Dr. Price.

Throughout the United States, food growers currently do not have to disclose whether or not a food contains GM ingredients. The American consumer is intentionally left uninformed about the food they eat. Many GM seeds have been banned from use in the European Union due to safety concerns. However, US growers are free to use them without differentiating which ingredients are genetically modified.

Four major GM food crops in the U.S. — soy, corn, canola and cotton — have been inserted with bacterial genes.
The majority of processed food products Americans eat daily contain some form of soybean, corn, canola (rapeseed) oil or cottonseed oil. If your food comes in a box from the supermarket, it is probably genetically engineered. The four crops listed in Figure 15 are used in vegetable oil. Other foods known to be genetically modified are papaya, rice, tomatoes, rapeseed, potatoes, sugar beets and peas.

Crop (% is GMO)	Products commonly containing GMOs
Soy (94%)*	Chocolates, breads, shakes, baby formulas
Cotton (93%)*	Chips, fried snack products
Canola (90%)*	Fried products, baked goods, many health products
Corn (88%)*	High fructose corn syrup found in sodas, cereals, cookies, candy, salad dressings, spaghetti sauces, cornstarch, breads and 10,000 other products

*Percentage of GM cotton, corn and soy in the U.S.; GM canola is grown in Canada
Source: Institute for Responsible Technology

Figure 15. Top GMO crops.

The best resource for learning more about the prevalence of GM foods is *Seeds of Deception* by Jeffrey M. Smith. His organization recommends buying produce labeled 100% organic or non-GMO, and avoiding the consumption of "at risk" ingredients from soy, corn, canola or cottonseed sources. When visiting your local farmer's markets, check with the farmer for their seed sources, and ask if they use GM seeds. Join a local community-supported agriculture (CSA) network of individuals who pledge to support local farms where growers and consumers share the risks and benefits of food production. CSA members pay at the onset of the growing season for a share of the anticipated harvest; once harvesting begins, they receive weekly shares of vegetables and fruit in a box, and sometimes herbs, cut flowers, honey, eggs, dairy products and meat.

When Mary Shelley published her book, *Frankenstein* in 1818, it was considered a work of science fiction. It is a story about scientist Victor Frankenstein and his creation — a creature with all the physiological features of a human, but larger and blemished. As the creature grows older, he wreaks havoc on the life of his creator, forcing Victor into a life of emotional turmoil, physical trauma and ultimately death.

The creation of genetically modified organisms is no longer science fiction — it is science fact. Biotech companies, such as Monsanto, have created them under the auspices of the FDA and Environmental Protection Agency (EPA). The physical and biological impacts these organisms have had and will have on the health of the human population have not been thoroughly tested. There are no measures to guarantee that the GM Frankensteins of our time will not cause our deaths. Dr. Harvey Wiley was the last stalwart within the FDA who spent his life attempting to thwart the grotesque manipulation of nature's perfect foods. Without a successor to follow in his footsteps, each and every one of us must increase our personal commitment to consume only organic, non-GMO whole foods. Furthermore, as an added benefit, not consuming any processed food will automatically lower the risk of consuming the four major GMO crops. We must also hold food manufacturers accountable for honest labeling of any food that contains GMO. Lastly, we must continue to support our local farmer's markets and CSAs, and become growers of food in our very own backyards.

MODERN DAY HEALTH CRUSADER

In November 2012, there was an epic battle to ensure honest and truthful reporting on food labels in California. Proposition 37 was started by a grandmother in Chico, California who wanted to do something about the unabated proliferation of genetically engineered foods and the resultant huge increase in the use of pesticides. She started a grassroots movement and recruited many people in support. Local organic farmers and organic produce companies supported increasing awareness and the need for truthful labeling.

Unfortunately, many biotechnology and chemical companies, including Monsanto, funded the opposition of Proposition 37 with the use of blitz television marketing. With over 50% of the company's revenues generated from the sale of GM seeds, they opposed this measure that could potentially educate all consumers on the widespread presence of GM foods.[136] The San Jose Mercury News reported:

"St. Louis-based Monsanto, a leading producer of genetically engineered seeds and chemicals such as the herbicide Roundup, has donated $4.2 million to efforts to defeat Proposition 37"[137]

The money donated to the campaign in support of Proposition 37 came from many small organic food companies. The largest financial supporter of Proposition 37 lives outside of California. He knew it was important to increase the awareness of food safety across the nation. His name is Dr. Joseph Mercola.

Dr. Mercola has been a licensed physician and surgeon in the state of Illinois since 1982. In 1997, he established www.mercola.com, which is now the world's #1 ranked natural health website, with over a million newsletter subscribers. His purpose is to transform the prevailing medical paradigm by empowering everybody with honest information. His goal is to educate and support the optimization of health through proper nutrition, coupled with exercise and good, natural lifestyle choices.

Even though Proposition 37 did not pass, it set a precedent. The sheer voice of thousands of Californians who voted for the Proposition is indicative that consumers still want the right to know where their food originates. Furthermore, Proposition 37 was iconic because it demonstrated that while many individuals are strong enough to stand up for themselves, we also stand together with those who are strong enough to stand up for others. As health crusaders in the making, we must all demand healthy food for real people.

Question #4 to ask your holistic health care practitioner:
Do you stay abreast with the information provided on Dr. Joseph Mercola's website?

12

SYNTHETIC VITAMINS DO
NOT DO A BODY GOOD

"The whole is more than the sum of its parts."

— Aristotle

During junior high school, I read about neurotransmitters and how specific amino acids from protein, minerals and other nutrients serve as precursors to their formation. Neurotransmitters are hormones that transmit signals from a neuron to another across a synapse, the space between nerve cells. Our brain requires neurotransmitters to facilitate proper nerve firing, the formation of memories, and logical thinking. In preparation for my college entrance exams, the SATs, I searched for supplements to enhance my cognitive abilities and elevate my IQ. I did not know that most of the supplements I purchased from local health food stores contained synthetic vitamins and isolated nutrients. Some of the "brain powders" I consumed even contained aspartame, an artificial sweetener used as an ant poison. Many of my friends and family have also turned to supplements hoping to use nutrition as medicine. However, many of these products do very little to feed our bodies — and may even cause harm.

The growing "nutraceutical" industry gives rise to a market filled with laboratory-made imitations that are now concentrated and dosed similar to pharmaceuticals in order to create pharmacological effects. A nutraceutical is a nutrient-like drug marketed under the blurred umbrella of "nutrition." Unfortunately, nutraceutical marketers are neglecting to inform consumers that vitamins, minerals and other nutrients from whole foods have and always will be the best form of nutrition for humans. Why would they want to remind you of that?

Nutraceuticals are big business. Sales of supplements, made primarily from synthetic and isolated nutrients, totaled $50.4 billion in 2010 in the US and continues to grow.[138] Most synthetic vitamins are made by five pharmaceutical companies and then rebranded under hundreds of different labels. Centrum®, one of the largest synthetic vitamin lines, is owned and marketed by Pfizer, the largest pharmaceutical company on the planet.[tt]

High dose synthetic vitamin supplements are purported to work due to the pharmacological effect on the body — which is not the same as the nutritional effect. No whole food ever contained a high amount of a few select nutrients. For example, ascorbic acid (which the FDA allows food manufacturers to claim as Vitamin C) works well in acute infections, but can be toxic when taken long-term in high doses. Any high dosed synthetic or isolated vitamin taken long-term can lead to weakened health because the body always expects nutrients from whole food sources. Judith Decava's *The Real Truth about Vitamins and Anti-oxidants* states, "synthetic thiamine (Thiamine HCL or Thiamine Mononitrate), will initially allay fatigue but will eventually cause fatigue by the buildup of pyruvic acid. This leads to the vicious cycle of thinking more and more thiamine is

---

[tt] Bayer Healthcare, besides aspirin, markets the One A Day® and Flintstones Kids™ vitamin lines. Otsuka America Pharmaceuticals Inc. owns Nature's Resource vitamin line. GlaxoSmithKline, Johnson & Johnson, Alcon, Bausch & Lomb and Novartis also have a large presence in the synthetic vitamin markets.

needed, resulting in more and more fatigue along with other accumulated complaints... Natural food-source vitamins are enzymatically alive. Man-made synthetic vitamins are dead chemicals."

As I studied for the SATs, I took a synthetic B vitamin supplement to counteract the extreme fatigue from studying hundreds of four syllable words and practicing endless analogue and critical reading exercises. Perhaps all the naps I took in between were due to the fatigue caused by a thiamine HCl overdose. It is difficult to know. I also wonder if my SAT scores were negatively influenced by high dosage synthetic supplements. Furthermore, did I create long-term harm to my body?

Whole food sourced vitamins are far superior to the counterfeits or imitations that laboratories concoct from a base of chemicals. Clinical studies show that administering one fraction of a food nutrient or a synthetic version of it can have disappointing or even toxic results, some noxious enough to increase the risk of cancer, heart disease, stroke and disease of all sorts.[139,140] How come this information is never included on synthetic vitamin supplement labels? In order for those manufacturers to earn a profit, they rely on you to believe that synthetic vitamins are just as nourishing to the healing body as whole food. This is fact: humans cannot outsmart nature. So it is important to know how synthetic vitamins are harmful in high dosages.

HIGH DOSE SYNTHETICS = PHARMACOLOGY

A friend and colleague, who has been studying holistic healing modalities for decades, has a library filled with reference books on how foods heal the body and how pharmaceutical products hamper its processes. I stumbled across a book on how pharmaceutical medications induce nutrient depletion. In that moment I asked myself, "Could anything made by a pharmaceutical company actually address a nutritional deficiency?"

Intuitively, I knew it was impossible, but I wanted to understand why. As I glanced over my friend's library, I found a few books documenting the history of vitamins — methods of discovery and how the pharmaceutical industry learned to create synthetic versions. And then I asked myself, "What is a synthetic vitamin? Can they be harmful to our health?"

What I found was evidence that synthetic vitamins lack essential co-factors, which complete and balance the whole nutrient complex. Whole food sources contain all related nutrients — vitamins, minerals, trace elements, enzymes, coenzymes, amino acids, fatty acids and unidentified factors — that function together in the physiology of the body. When single vitamins are supplemented with separated fractions or synthetic chemicals, the effect is unwholesome and can lead to depletion and imbalance.[141,142]

The term "wholesome" refers to a complete food in its natural and unrefined state. For example, the entire Vitamin A complex is composed of the active Vitamin A, retinol palmitate, and over 600 known carotenoids. Unfortunately, synthetic vitamins often supply a high dosage of one, two or even three of the known 600. Each year, scientists are discovering new carotenoids in whole foods, which are required by the body for proper functioning. The most common synthetic "Vitamin A" is beta-carotene. Swiss pharmaceutical company, Hoffman-LaRoche produces most of the world's supply. In one manufacturing plant alone, they produce 350 tons each year.[143] This form cannot be converted to the active Vitamin A, retinol palmitate, because the other nutrients that accompany it in whole foods are no longer included.

Similarly, the entire Vitamin E complex is made up of tocopherols (delta, gamma, beta, alpha), tocotrienols (delta, gamma, beta, alpha), xanthine, selenium, lipositols, E2 factor, E3 factor, F1 factor and F2 factor. See Figure 16. Unfortunately, the FDA has allowed companies to label alpha-tocopherol as Vitamin E. However, the function of alpha-tocopherol is to serve as an anti-oxidant protector to the nutrients in the entire Vitamin E complex. While there are studies demonstrating the pharmacological use of alpha-tocopherol or isolated components of the Vitamin E complex in high dosages, many more demonstrate its dangers. High dosages of alpha-tocopherol have been known to cause nausea, flatulence, diarrhea,

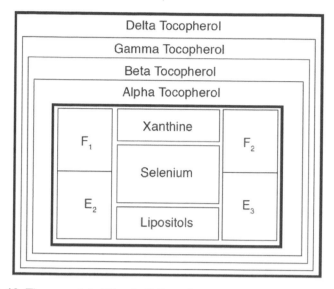

Figure 16. The complete Vitamin E Complex.

increased heart failure and cardiovascular mortality due to left ventricular dysfunction.[144],[145] Growth retardation, poor bone calcification, reduced hematocrit (alteration of healthy red blood cells) levels and reduced skeletal muscle respiration have also been reported in animal studies.[146,147,148] The incidence of retinitis pigmentosa (night blindness) increases when a person takes high dosages of alpha-tocopherol combined with high dosage of synthetic vitamin A.[149]

The best source of the whole Vitamin E complex in the proportion that nature has always packaged it is wheat germ oil. The body inherently knows what to do with a whole food source of the Vitamin E complex. Conversely, alpha-tocopherol is an isolate that causes additional stress on the body by forcing it to physiologically compensate for missing factors.

The entire Vitamin B complex includes over 25 members. The most studied are thiamin (B_1), riboflavin (B_2), niacinamide (B_3), pyridoxine (B_6), cyanocobalamin (B_{12}), biotin, choline, inositol, pantothenic acid, folic acid and para-aminobenzoic acid (PABA). Excellent food sources of these are organ meats (such as liver), brewer's yeast, whole grains (especially from bran and germ), nuts, beans and peas. They are essential to all cells for energy production. All preparations of single B vitamins or even of several single B vitamin (combined in so-called "high potency") supplements are synthetic, chemically isolated, altered and unnatural in form. In some cases, the synthetic forms are completely unusable. For example, synthetic Vitamin B_1, commonly listed as thiamine hydrochloride or thiamine mononitrate, is very different from the natural form the body uses. Biochemist Dr. Albert L. Lehninger found that the human body cannot properly metabolize and utilize the synthetic forms of Vitamin B_1 because they cannot be phosphorylated into the usable carboxylase or thiamine pyrophosphate, which are essential to the production of pyruvic acid, needed for glucose degradation in the mitochondrial Krebs (citric acid) cycle.[150]

Synthetic Vitamin B_1 is known to be biochemically unusable by the body — and it is extremely toxic in large doses. At 10 milligrams or more per day, there have been reports of edema, shaking, tremors, nervousness, disturbances in heart rhythms, severe disturbances in heart and nerve function, tachycardia (change in heart rate), fatty liver and decreased blood pressure.

Dr. Barnett Sure at University of Arkansas Department of Agriculture Chemistry found synthetic thiamine hydrochloride to cause sterility and infertility in animal subjects — sounds like a "neuter"-ceutical to me.[151]

Many consumers think to reach for a high dose of ascorbic acid (erroneously referred to as Vitamin C) during times of illness or immune challenge. In acute situations it will work pharmacologically, but using it long-term can create other health hazards.‡

In the early 1930s, Albert Szent-Györgyi isolated and identified one portion of Vitamin C, the ascorbic acid component (see Figure 17). This was a huge discovery, for generations of sailors and city dwellers were afflicted with scurvy, bleeding gums and other Vitamin

---

‡ Short-term use of high dose ascorbic acid lowers the pH of the blood below 7.4 which temporarily prevents pathogenic bacteria from flourishing. Long-term pharmacologic alterations of blood pH may fatigue the lungs and kidney organs which maintain blood pH homeostasis.

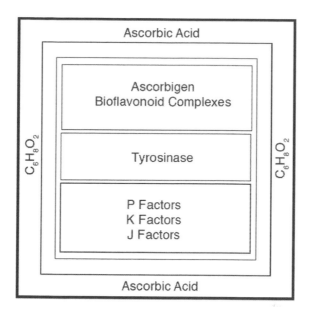

Figure 17. The complete Vitamin C Complex.

C-deficient illnesses. He instantly became a candidate for a Nobel Prize. He shared his results with pharmaceutical companies and they began to synthetically manufacture ascorbic acid, which they began marketing as Vitamin C in 1934.

Szent-Györgyi, wanting to confirm his findings that ascorbic acid was the active constituent of Vitamin C, conducted additional studies. He found that the bioflavanoids, originally called Vitamin P, from lemons or red pepper were actually the nutrients responsible for clearing up a hemorrhagic condition even when pure ascorbic acid from some other source was useless. He describes it as:

> *"The active substance (Vitamin P) was found in the end in a fraction consisting of practically pure flavone or flavonal glycoside. Forty milligrams of this fraction given daily intravenously to man restored in a fortnight regularly the normal capillary resistance. Spontaneous bleeding ceased, the capillary walls lost their fragility towards pressure differences and no more plasma protein left the vascular system on increased venous pressure."*[152]

Szent-Györgyi and his team went on to discover in 1935 that the entire Vitamin C complex included bioflavonoids (Vitamin P and Vitamin J), ascorbigen, tyrosinase and K factors. He returned to the Nobel Assembly to inform them that his discovery of ascorbic acid was not the complete and active part of the whole Vitamin C complex. Unfortunately, the commercial industry had already begun mass production of ascorbic acid and began selling it as Vitamin C. Hoffmann LaRoche became the first company to mass-produce synthetic ascorbic acid in 1934. More than 90% of ascorbic acid in the U.S. is manufactured in their Nutley, New Jersey manufacturing plant.

Today, many high-dose synthetic and isolated vitamins are derived from coal tar, petroleum and corn syrup from genetically modified corn. When was the last time you had a petroleum or coal tar deficiency?

Question #5 to ask your holistic health care practitioner:
Are you aware that the use of synthetic vitamins in high dosages is pharmacology?

Food for Thought: Most retail supplements contain high doses of synthetic vitamins. If you see Vitamin C is listed as ascorbic acid, it is most likely synthetic based. If you see Vitamin E listed as alpha-tocopherols (and not from pea vine juice or wheat germ oil), it is most likely synthetic based. If you see Vitamin A listed as beta-carotene, it is most likely synthetic based. If you see multiple vitamins listed, claiming to provide over a hundred percent of Daily Value, it is most likely derived from synthetic materials as well. Furthermore, the nutrients within a product are most likely not derived from food sources if the supplement label does not list multiple food sources. Supplements that contain artificial colorings are almost always synthetic based and should be avoided.

PLANTS EAT ROCKS

When I was a child, I often went to the park to play with my relatives. One day, I watched my younger cousin rolling in the dirt, doing somersaults and cartwheels, creating a cloud of dust. As her older cousin, I warned, "Stop rolling in the dirt. Your mom and dad are gonna be mad."

She continued to run yelling, "God made dirt and dirt don't hurt." Then she grabbed some dirt and chewed it for three seconds when out came a rock, followed by whatever she could spit out. My insight: humans should not eat dirt and absolutely avoid eating rocks.

Unfortunately, many mineral supplement products are laboratory chelated or made from finely ground rocks that our bodies were not designed to consume. Chelation binds a mineral to a protein for transport into and out of our bodies. Supplement companies with commercial interests have wanted us to believe that calcium, regardless of the source, is always usable by our bodies. Unfortunately, that is far from the truth.

Our bodies are designed to use calcium in the form of calcium bicarbonate, which is typically found in naturally occurring spring water but immediately converts to calcium carbonate when exposed to air. For our body to use calcium carbonate it must undergo twelve enzymatic reactions to convert into usable calcium bicarbonate. Each of the enzymatic reactions requires various trace minerals, vitamins, and nutrients, which could tax an already nutritionally starved body.

Most synthetic mineral supplements contain calcium carbonate, usually coral from the ocean or limestone (rock). A better form for our body is calcium citrate, found in eggshells, and calcium lactate, found in mother's breast milk and fermented vegetables such as beets. Calcium citrate requires three enzymatic reactions within the body for utilization, and calcium lactate requires only one, which makes it the easiest form to assimilate.

When we use high dose supplements extracted from rocks or artificially chelated in labs, we create mineral imbalances and wreak havoc on the body's detoxifying organs because unconverted rock or pharmaceutical-based minerals must exit the body. Unfortunately, as

Dr. Melvin Page found whole food nutrition relies heavily on the preservation of balanced mineral ratios.

No scientist will ever be capable of creating a synthetic supplement which duplicates the ratios of minerals found in whole food sources. Nature knows best. Plants have a method of extracting minerals from the soil. They eat the rocks and chelate them into a form that humans and animals can consume, digest, assimilate and use. Animals eat these plants and then humans eat the animals or the plants directly to obtain these minerals. The bioavailability of minerals from natural whole food sources is greater than from isolated vitamins, inorganic mineral salts or mineral chelates.[153,154, 155]

The best mineral sources are bone broths, dark green leafy vegetables, alfalfa sprouts and seaweeds such as kelp. Eat your vegetables, seaweeds and bone broths, and leave the rocks in the dirt.

THE LIFE FORCE OF FOOD

The main difference between a supplement with high dosages of synthetically made nutrients and raw whole food concentrates is the life force they contain. Whole food concentrates are essentially raw food in a tablet, and are energetically alive. In Traditional Chinese Medicine, nourishing foods are known to have "Gu Qi" (穀氣), which means "energy of living foods."

Synthetic chemicals lack life and actually drain the body's reserves. Claiming that the ascorbic acid made in a lab has the same molecular chemistry as that found in food is like saying a living being has the same cellular makeup as a fresh corpse. Vitamin complexes are so biochemically complicated that only a living cell can create them. Just as a computer programmer will never recreate a human brain, chemists will never reproduce a true vitamin in a laboratory.

Dr. Royal Lee explained that vitamins are biological mechanisms. "Like a watch, they consist of a multitude of parts — some we may never identify — that act together to deliver to the body a transcendent 'vitamin effect.' The chemist (and modern synthetic vitamin supplement maker) who isolates a few parts of a vitamin complex and expects these parts to deliver the effect of the entire mechanism might as well slap a few pieces of brass on his or her wrist and ask them to tell time."

Reductionist chemists and biochemists believe that nutritional complexes can be reduced to, or at least approximated by, their "most important" parts. To these critics, we ask, "Which part of a watch keeps time?" No single part, of course. The various pieces work together to perform a function that transcends that of any of the individual parts. Moreover, only the complete set of parts will perform the function. Remove just one of these parts, and the mechanism fails.

The whole food concentrates created by Dr. Lee contain every known nutrient. As scientists discover new nutrients each year, they find them to already be in Dr. Lee's formulas. It is impossible for a synthetic based supplement to provide us the nutrients that have not yet been discovered. While science has a long way to catch up to nature, we don't have to wait to feed our bodies the foods we were designed to eat.

<u>Question #6 to ask your holistic health care practitioner:</u>
Are you trained in how to use the whole food concentrates created by Dr. Royal Lee?

13

EMPTY HARVEST

"To get the iron that was available in 1 cup of spinach in 1945, you would have to consume 65 cups today."

— Any top soil expert

Billy walked into my clinic for his afternoon follow-up appointment. At the beginning of his nutritional evaluation, I asked, "How was your lunch?"

He responded confidently, "I had a spinach salad."

I smiled and then inquired for more detail, "Did you eat 65 salads?" Since our conversation took place 66 years after 1945, I was concerned about his body receiving a sufficient amount of iron and other nutrients. I could have asked him if he had traveled back 66 years to eat that salad in his time machine. But since he arrived fifteen minutes late for his appointment, I figured time travel was a slim possibility.

Unfortunately, Billy didn't know that the nutritional content of most vegetables and foods we eat today is far less than what our grandparents ate. Because of this, Billy and most Americans are undernourished. We are nutritionally starving, not from an insufficient quantity of food, but due to deficiencies of nutrients in food. Soil depletion, air pollution, water pollution, toxin and pollution elevation, sub-par modern farming methods, crop limitation, overutilization of fields, and food refining and processing have escalated since the 1960s. They have become exponentially worse in the present day. Plants and vegetables grown for human consumption are not what they used to be.

Most all vitamins in food are either directly or indirectly produced by plants. The exceptions are Vitamin D, which can be produced by body exposure to the ultraviolet light from the sun, and Vitamin B12, which is produced by fungi, soil microorganisms (actinomycetes) and some bacteria in our small and large intestines. The beneficial bacteria that reside in our intestines normally produce a portion of our Vitamin K needs, as well as smaller quantities of some other B complex vitamins. Nutrient dense foods are still — and always will be — the only source of virtually all the vitamins, minerals and nutrients our bodies need. The quality of the soil determines the nutrient density of all foods. Soils must rest, revive and regenerate with fresh, organic compost to maintain a rich biodiversity. Healthy soil gives rise to nutrient dense plant life. Healthy plants provide nourishing foods for animals and humans. Minerals, both macro and micro (trace), are so important for our health that we can no longer overlook how we are being robbed nutritionally by conventional and commercial farmers.

MACRO AND MICRO MINERALS

During my freshman year at U.C. Berkeley, I had a roommate who delivered my early teachings on the basics of agriculture. An herbalist, he had to properly formulate the right soil mixture to grow strong herbs that he could one day pack into a pipe or bong, a device for extracting the active constituents of home grown cannabis. He discussed the importance of nitrogen, phosphorous and potassium (known from the periodic table as NPK). His soil required sufficient amounts of these minerals in the proper ratio to grow quickly, be strong and develop a rich dark green color. I learned that Baron Justus von Liebig, had published articles in the 1840s, indicating that only these three minerals were needed. Synthetically feeding these to plants, farmers could force them to support the vegetable consumption of an increasing human population. From this theory published in 1855 as *Agricultural Chemistry*, the agriculture industry exploded with the widespread use of *"artificial manure"* and synthetic fertilizers.

Since Liebig's NPK theory, it has been confirmed that plants also require secondary nutrients (calcium, magnesium and sulfur) and trace minerals to grow strong and healthy. The trace minerals required in small quantities are boron, copper, iron, manganese, selenium, molybdenum, iodine and zinc. Coincidentally, our endocrine system requires a constant intake of these trace minerals for proper glandular function. For example, copper consumed from whole food sources feeds the bones, skin and adrenal glands; iodine supports the thyroid, breast, uterine and prostate tissues; manganese feeds the pituitary and joints; zinc the prostate, uterus and liver. However, the commercial focus of large-scale agriculture is to grow plants and vegetables rapidly to sell at the market. Unfortunately, many farmers overlook the necessity of replenishing trace minerals in the topsoil. Years after Liebig brought forward the NPK theory, a German naturalist named Julius Hensel stated that if farmers spread finely crushed, mineral rich rock dust onto their farmlands to restore minerals on depleted soil, they would, "be amazed at the quality, strength, and drought resistance of their crops."

We as consumers cannot measure the trace minerals in our foods with the naked eye. We rarely know about the quality of soils in which our produce was grown. We usually rely on our eyesight and sense of smell to assess the freshness of produce we purchase. But this provides little information on the nutritional content. To know the quality of our food, we need to build relationships with our farmers — to learn whether they farm merely for profit by only focusing on NPK to ensure rapid growth, or if they understand that farming begins by building the health and vitality of soil filled with trace minerals to grow food that nourishes the healing body.

Although my college roommate never bothered to restore the trace mineral content in the soil he grew his herbs from, he did have multiple harvests to bake batches of brownies with. While they were most likely deficient in various trace minerals, he claimed they contained sufficient levels of the "other" nutrients for recreational use.

NOURISHING THE SOIL

The immune systems of humans and plants both depend on soil quality. To understand nutrition, one must become a farmer and learn what constitutes as a high quality soil. William Albrecht, Ph.D. at the University of Missouri confirmed that soil is a living substance. He found that he could cure livestock of undulant fever by feeding them nutrient dense food grown from soil infused with trace minerals. He also showed that plants were vulnerable to insects, fungi and other diseases when the soils lacked adequate minerals or contained toxic substances. When a tree develops an infection, the best and only natural method of remedying it is to feed the soil, which in turn feeds the tree's internal systems. Similarly when humans develop an infection, the optimal method of fighting it is to feed the body the proper nutrition, which bolsters the immune system's natural killer cells, macrophages and lymphocytes to restore homeostasis (balance). Well nourished soil will give rise to well nourished plants, that provide nutrient dense foods for animals and humans.

Dr. Royal Lee grew up practicing animal husbandry on his home farm. He learned by just altering the diet of a sick animal with increased amounts of specific high nutrient dense foods, he could support rapid healing. He maintained journals on effective food quantities, down to the milligram. His approach is how thousands of holistic health care practitioners support their patients today.

I have planted many fruit trees in my backyard, including a peach tree. One spring it showed signs of a fungal infection. The local nursery employees suggested immediate action by spraying a fungicide on the infected leaves. I wanted to consume chemical free peaches that next summer. Instead of topical fungicide spray, I fed the peach tree the most nutritious plant and tree food — an organic "compost tea" made by the worms in my composting bin. Within two weeks the fungal infection disappeared. This demonstrates that nourishing the soil will strengthen a plant from the inside to appear healthier on the outside. This also is true for animals and humans. Feed the body what it needs on the inside and the appearance of skin, hair and nails will improve.

Compost and organic material introduce beneficial microorganisms into the soil's complexity. Microorganisms commonly found in soil and compost convert organic nitrogen into inorganic nitrogen, a process called mineralization. Plants then take up the nutrients released by this process. Compost contains an astonishing variety of microbes, many of which may be beneficial for controlling pathogens. Organic matter improves soil structure, resulting in a crumbly feel with improved water retention, air infiltration, and fertility. Microorganisms can also break down contaminants in the soil and water to components that pose less of an environmental hazard.

Nature provides everything for humans to live bountifully. If we nourish the soil that nourishes our food, we can produce foods that nourish our healing bodies. Unfortunately, the opposite is also true. If we focus on three minerals while poisoning our soils with pesticides, insecticides, herbicides, fungicides and other chemicals, we gradually poison our societies through undernourished and toxic foods. Bio-dynamic, permaculture and organic farming methods are strategies to halt the future use of all chemicals used in agriculture. The revival of nutrient rich soils will give rise to nourishing vegetables, healthy animals, and ultimately, healthy humans. The health of human populations depends on the health of the soil at the root level. Humans have mistakenly placed themselves at the top of the food chain. Actually, maggots are above us on the food chain, for once we die, the health of our fleshy corpse determines whether the maggots reap the benefits of a nourished body or one of nutritional deficiency. This fact describes the circle of life. There is no tiered hierarchy, but

rather a food circle which makes inseparable the soil and its microorganisms, maggots, insects, plants, animals and humans.

THE POISONS IN THE SOIL

The *Silent Spring* was instrumental in bringing
widespread awareness to the ill effects of many
chemical pesticides. In it, Rachel Carson catalogued
the short and long-term environmental impacts of
the indiscriminate spraying and application of DDT
in the US. It brought regulators and the general
public to question the logic of releasing large
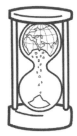
amounts of chemicals into the environment without fully
understanding their effects on ecology or human health. DDT was
banned in the US in 1972. Unfortunately, the movement requires
ongoing effort because commercial farmers continue to apply
chemical pesticides of other types to their land.

Pesticides are known to accumulate in the fat tissues of the body.
Mothers who consume produce from non-organic sources will
transfer these chemicals to their infants via breast milk. Pregnant
women also pass pesticides to their fetus in utero. In 2007,
approximately 33 million pounds of organophosphate pesticides were
sprayed on US farming soils. [156] Two of these, malathion and
chlorpyrifos, have been linked to cancer and neurological defects in
humans.[157,158,159] Despite their ban for home use, they are still used
commercially on a variety of crops in the US. Organophosphates
work by poisoning the nervous system of pests. Unfortunately, they
do the same in humans.[160] The research of Mark Purdey, an organic
dairy farmer in England, made clear that the Bovine Spongiform
Encephalopathy (BSE) epidemic, also known as mad cow disease, in
England occurred in areas where farmers were forced to treat their
cattle with organophosphates in a program to eradicate the warble
fly.[161]

Commercial farmers in the United States sprayed over 1.1 billion
pounds — 2% of the world's total pesticides — in 2007. There are

21,000 pesticide products containing 860 active ingredients. All are designed to kill living organisms, which is why the Environmental Protection Agency (EPA) prohibits claims that these chemicals are safe or nontoxic. The top ten pesticides applied in the agricultural market are glyphosate, atrazine, metolachlor-s, acetochlor, 2,4-dichlorophenoxyacetic acid and pendimethalin, plus the fumigants, metam sodium, dichloropropene, methyl bromide and chloropicrin. These are neurotoxic and known to cause cancer, birth defects, reproductive anomalies, liver and kidney damage and even death.[162,163,164,165,166,167] They also cause developmental and behavioral abnormalities as well as hormone and immune dysfunctions. The most documented pesticide is Agent Orange, a defoliant sprayed during the Vietnam War. Over 4.8 million Vietnamese were exposed to it leading to 400,000 deaths and disabilities, and half a million children born with birth defects. Monsanto is one of the manufacturers of Agent Orange, glyphosate and other herbicides.

Despite the toxicity of our farmlands, hope exists when we choose to consume foods grown organically and work with a holistic health care practitioner. A colleague of mine who is a licensed acupuncturist in Monterey County, CA, helped a 20-year-old man whose psychiatrist had diagnosed with bipolar disorder and prescribed an atypical antipsychotic drug for the management of symptoms. During my colleague's nutritional evaluation of the man, he discovered he had organophosphate toxicity impacting his fore-brain, cerebrospinal fluid, thyroid and adrenal glands. His mother reported when he was ten, his father had him help apply pesticides for hours. She remembered the incident vividly because he was hurrying to finish spraying so that he could attend a birthday party. Instead, syncopy, nausea and tremors sent him to the emergency room. The pesticides continued to impact this boy's life for over ten years. His reported "behavioral problems", including a brief brush with gang association, can perhaps be traced, in part, to that day. Fortunately, the acupuncturist provided an individualized nutritional program, including Dr. Lee's whole food concentrates to support his parotid, liver and adrenal glands. In just six months, he had detoxified the organophosphates out of his body, his bipolar symptoms disappeared, and his psychiatrist removed the bipolar medications from his program. He and his family are very excited about how whole food nutrition has helped him start a new life, healthy and un-medicated. Each and every one of us can live such a life.

Question #7 to ask your holistic health care practitioner:

Are you capable of identifying which organs are negatively impacted by pesticides or other chemicals and how to use whole food concentrates to support the body's ability to properly detoxify them out?

PART III:

A NEW HOPE

"Let food be thy medicine, and let thy medicine be thy food."

— Hippocrates

14

REGENERATE ORGANS

"吃什麼, 補什麼"
"Eat the organ which you want to fortify."

— A Chinese saying

During 2006-2008, I lived in Asia — a few months in Beijing and two years in Taipei for my Masters degree. During that time, I made many new friends and met distant relatives. Nearly every person I met in China and Taiwan knows the traditional wisdom that eating a particular organ will support your own organ's regeneration and function. Out of curiosity, I informally surveyed my friends and family to see which of them actually ate organ meats. Those born before 1960 still ate liver, kidneys, hearts and intestines on a regular basis. But the younger generation, accustomed to eating commercialized foods, seldom consumed organ meats, unless it was prepared by the older generation. Similarly, most Americans shriek or cringe at the idea of consuming organ meats.

Organ meats are an effective source of nutrition. Nutritional analysis confirms that liver is at the top of the list among the most nutrient dense foods. Dr. Price observed that native peoples traditionally consumed organ meats. The Inuit told him that the adrenal glands of a moose prevent scurvy. When a moose was killed, they immediately extracted the adrenal gland and its fat to be shared equally among all members of the tribe. The adrenal glands and walls of the second stomach of the moose indeed have high amounts of the whole Vitamin C complex.

ORGANOTHERAPY

The use of organ meats to support the restoration and regeneration of human organs is documented back to 500 B.C. in Indian, Hebrew and Arabic texts. In 2000 B.C., the Chinese *Materia Medica* by Shen Nong lists a diverse collection of remedies from animal, plant and mineral sources. Many of the foods used as medicine were consumed through the late 19th century. Even during the 1940s, glandular extracts were part of Western medicine.

In 1923, Dr. Brailsford Robertson, a professor at U.C. Berkeley, found that he could extract components to stimulate organ and cell growth. He discovered specific growth proteins, which he called *tethelin,* to be of great value for treating slow-healing wounds. He went on to discover the growth factor of the pituitary gland and showed that certain growth factors could be separated from every living cell to stimulate growth in a culture medium. The degree of concentration of the substance was significant in regulating growth.

Dr. Royal Lee invented equipment and machinery to extract and concentrate these specific components from organs and organ tissues. In the 1950s, he developed glandular products, which he called Protomorphogen™ extracts. These are not the usual desiccated glandulars, but are uniquely derived nucleoprotein-mineral extracts that support organ health at the cellular level.

Protomorphogen™ is derived from the Greek "proto" meaning primary and "morphogen" meaning form or structure of the initial element. It refers to the specific cytotrophic cellular material extracted from the cell nucleus containing the nucleoprotein. This contains the genetic DNA and RNA that regulates structural regeneration of the cell.[168] These chromosomal end products made in the cell nucleus are the agents or blueprints by which the basic functions of the chromosomes are exercised.

All living proteins carry a component which makes it specific in causing organic reactions, specific in function, and specific in its ability to act as an antigen in modulating immune reactions. The Protomorphogen™ formulations do not provide nutrients to the body, but rather provide genetic blueprints to reprogram the particular cell type to produce normal healthy cells.

The theory of protomorphology was derived from (and later verified by) the work of many other scientists around the world, such as Dr. Fenton B. Turck's "Cytost", M.T. Burrow's "Archusia/Ergusia", J.H. Northrup's "Proteinozen", G.W. Beadle's "Protogene", Mast and Pace's "X-substance", M.R. Drennan's "Biophores", Alexis Carrel's "Heat stable growth inhibitor" and Antoine Bechamp's "Mycrozyma" which all referred to the same elements discussed in the theory of protomorphology. These are just different names for the growth factors and blueprints of various living cells.

They are mineral chains whose sequencing determines the amino acid structure of individual cell types. In living tissues these minerals are organically bound and accompanied by enzymes. Modern allopathic medicine still does not understand how wounds are healed. What stimulates the need for repair? What stops the repair after it has been completed? The answers and tools are in the protomorphogens from whole food sources and our own cells.

A protomorphogen has two major functions: to control healthy cell growth and regulate immunity. The regulation and control of the growth and regeneration process is very complicated, involving all of the endocrine glands, especially the thyroid, pituitary, adrenal, thymus and spleen. In working with any illness, holistic health care practitioners may facilitate the balancing and rebuilding of these endocrine glands and other organs with the use of Protomorphogen™ extracts and whole food concentrates.

In numerous lectures and writings, Dr. Royal Lee explained the complex interrelationships between immune response, normal and abnormal cell growth, and autoimmunity. He formulated concentrates of animal derived products that could normalize and balance the immune system and virtually every organ in the human body. A detailed explanation of the theory and application is well charted and explored in his book, *Applied Protomorphology*.

> **Food for Thought:** Stem cell research is and always will remain an ethical debate because of the involvement of embryonic tissues. To date, millions of dollars have been spent to develop a medicine that will enable doctors to inject substances that support the regeneration of various organs and glands. Voters and legislators are in a constant debate about whether more funds should be invested in such research. The desired application of stem cells is to regenerate organs. There is already a community of healers who are helping patients regenerate organs with the use of whole food nutrition, herbs, acupuncture and chiropractic care.

SHRINKAGE BY HORMONES

One day during my freshman year in high school, after P.E. class, a classmate asked me if I thought all baseball players or just those who were breaking home run records used exogenous testosterone and other anabolic steroids. I told him I didn't know who was juicing and who wasn't. I shrugged, "I guess you could check the size of their testicles. If they're small, then they must be using steroids."

"Is that how they test for it?" He was incredulous.

Even as teenagers, we knew that ball players took steroids to build muscle mass, increase speed and enhance strength. We also heard that the side effects included shrinking of the testicles. We always wondered how small they could shrink. Would they become the size of a pea or raisin? Would they shrink even more if cold water was added into the mix? Neither of us knew why or how this happened.

When athletes or body builders inject anabolic steroids, usually testosterone, their testicles have been shown to shrink because they are no longer required to produce and secrete testosterone into the blood stream. [169] The hypothalamus gland functions to release Gonadotropin-Releasing Hormone (GnRH) to stimulate the pituitary gland to produce and secrete luteinizing hormone (LH). In turn, the pituitary signals the testicles to produce and release testosterone (see Figure 18). If there is already too much testosterone in the blood stream due to the testosterone injection, none of this is needed and the hypothalamus involutes (shrinks). The pituitary receives a negative feedback message to decrease the release of LH, which lessens the stimulation of the testicles. The pituitary gland itself begins to shrink, but we cannot see it because it is located deep at the base of the brain. [170]

All hormone replacement therapy — whether synthetic, bio-identical, or xeno (foreign) in origin — prevents a person's own glands from regenerating to a point where they can produce hormones when the body needs them. Most medical doctors and non-holistic health care practitioners who prescribe exogenous (from outside of the body) hormones almost always overdose the patient, which leads to the suppression and subsequent weakening of their endocrine glands.

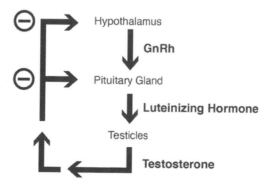

Figure 18. Negative Feedback Loop Mechanism of Testosterone.

The reaction of involution also occurs in people who are prescribed thyroid hormones like Synthroid® which contains the synthetic version of the thyroid hormone, thyroxine (also known as T4). Allopathic medical doctors dose patients on Synthroid® to the point that pituitary gland suppression occurs. One function, among many, of the pituitary gland is to regulate thirst and dryness of the mouth, so many patients who are overdosed on pituitary suppressing medications may develop thirst irregularities and other pituitary gland health challenges. Synthroid® also prevents the thyroid from regenerating, because the thyroid gland is no longer required to produce endogenous (of the body) thyroxine (T4) hormone, just as exogenous testosterone causes the testicles to stop hormone production and shrink.

Exogenous hormones impact the gland responsible for producing that particular hormone, which inhibits its regeneration. For example, the beta-cells in the pancreas will not be able to fully regenerate while a patient is undertaking insulin therapy. Furthermore, synthetic cortisol-based medications, such as prednisone prevent the adrenals from gaining strength.

With the use of organotherapy and whole food concentrates, it is possible to restore optimal glandular function so that sufficient quantities of needed hormones can be produced by the body itself. Men who have taken anabolic steroids are still able to restore hormonal balance and return their testicles to a healthy state. Women who have been declared infertile by an allopathic medical doctor can start cycling regularly and eventually conceive with the use of whole food concentrates. Those with thyroid hormone imbalances can restore their thyroid gland so that hormone replacement therapies are no longer required.

DON'T RIP MY ORGAN OUT

I recall the first girl I fell in love with. She had eyes that sparkled from a mile away, hair that shone like silk, and a smile that made my heart melt. Her teeth were extremely straight, which I now suspect was due to eating organ meats similar to native people — but more

Case Study – Restoring Fertility Naturally

A colleague who is a Doctor of Chiropractic in San Jose, CA advised a patient who was diagnosed with "ovarian failure" by her allopathic medical doctor. The patient and her husband had tried for over a year to conceive a second child with no success. After three months of nutritional upgrades, along with specific whole food concentrates to regenerate her liver, ovary and pituitary glands, her period returned and in five months she became pregnant. The goal after her pregnancy was to continue her nutritional program and chiropractic care to continue improving her health for the sake of her baby's health. She gave birth to a healthy baby and had no problems breastfeeding for two years. Today my colleague is the entire family's primary care doctor. They are all healthy and un-medicated.

likely attributed to excellent orthodontic care. Even though we attended the same English class, I never had the confidence to ask her for her phone number, let alone help proofreading my papers. Although I caught glimpses of her in the dining commons, I never said a word to her, not even a smile to indicate my interest. A few years after we graduated, I was formally introduced to her by a mutual friend. On our first date, a spark was lit. We spoke on the phone for hours at a time and it felt like I had known her for years. Then one evening, we sat in my car.

She told me she would be moving to the East Coast for graduate school. In the background, Paul Young's single "Every Time You Go Away" was playing on the radio.

"Can't you see, we've got everything goin' on and on and on,
Every time you go away, you take a piece of me with you…"

I was happy to hear she had been accepted at Harvard, but I was not interested in a long distance relationship. As I drove home, I decided to leave my job and move to Boston for her. I planned on calling her the next day to share the news.

But before I could call, she sent me an email saying we should break it off. I called her and left a voicemail. She responded to my message by email. So I emailed back, asking why. She too, believed that long distance relationships are unsuccessful most of the time. I wrote back that I would move to Boston, but she instructed me to stay in California — she did not want to be obligated to stay in a relationship that wouldn't work out.

I was crushed. She had ripped my heart to shreds. I realized an unbridled and innocent love could be vibrant and alive one day, but fall into shambles the next. The emotional pain was excruciating, as if someone had ripped out my heart with a knife, diced it into cubes and thrown it to the seagulls that feed on the bleachers after a baseball game.

Unfortunately, surgeons literally cut out patients' organs and throw them away every day, while assuming there are no long-term emotional or physical implications. Even worse, by not replacing removed organs demonstrates that surgeons deem them no longer important or even necessary.

Each year:

- Over 700,000 cholecystectomies (gallbladder removals) are performed.[171]
- Nearly 600,000 tonsillectomies (lymph tissue removals) are performed.[172]
- Over 600,000 hysterectomies (uterus and/or ovary removals§§) are performed.[173]
- Over 400,000 prostatectomies (prostate removals) are performed.[174]
- Many splenectomies (spleen removals) and thyroidectomies (thyroid removals) are performed.

There are times when surgical removal of an organ is completely necessary. More often than not, however, an organ's inability to regenerate merely indicates a long-standing nutritional deficiency,

§§ Some refer to a hysterectomy as female castration.

resulting in chronic dysfunction. Removing an organ without the replacement of a healthy substitute is blatant neglect by the allopathic profession. The removed organs served multiple vital functions for that person. The spleen aids in the maturation and storage of red blood cells, lymphocytes, monocytes and platelets, assists in wound healing and maintains normal calcium levels in the blood. Without a spleen, the body has difficulties performing these functions. The thyroid regulates metabolism, growth and body temperature. The gallbladder stores bile and releases it to help with the emulsification of fat, assimilation of fat-soluble nutrients, normalcy of bowel movements and prevention of bacterial infections. The tonsils support the fighting of infections, drainage of toxins and transport of white blood cells between lymph nodes and bone marrow. Unfortunately, most allopathic medical doctors lack the information and nutritional tools to help a person's body regenerate organs and restore their normal and healthy functions. Gallbladder, spleen, thyroid, uterus, ovary and prostate removals are not necessary when proper nutrition is implemented and no evidence of physical trauma is present.

Organ removals lead to worsened states of malnutrition. The removal of a gallbladder with no transplantation of a replacement causes patients to insufficiently emulsify fats and poorly assimilate fat-soluble nutrients like Vitamins A, D, E, K and F. After a gallbladder is removed, what will prevent the rest of the body from deteriorating from systemic fat-soluble nutrient deficiencies? Patients must ask their medical doctors about this prior to gallbladder removal.

Before you decide to have an organ removed, research the potential long-term symptoms. If you are already missing an organ, your holistic health care practitioner will be able to provide you with the proper whole food concentrates to fill the anatomical and physiological gaps your surgeon created. My heart was ripped apart, but it eventually healed. In time, it even became strong again and my willingness to interact with the members of the opposite sex was fully restored. As Tennyson wrote, "It is better to have loved and lost, than never to have loved at all." Emotionally, I experienced the blissful transcendence of love, survived the emotional pain of its loss and recovered with a humbled heart.

Physically, each one of our organs has the ability to heal, regenerate and become strong again. However, this only remains true if they are allowed to remain within our bodies. In order to keep our organs healthy enough so they never require removal, we must feed them early and feed them well. A holistic health care practitioner who implements whole food nutrition can support us to do so. It is my dream — a possible one — that we become collectively healthy so that we can sing Paul Young's song, with slightly modified lyrics for our allopathic medical doctors:

"Every time you go away, please DON'T take a piece of me with you..."

Question #1 to ask yourself:
Who is my holistic health care practitioner?

Case Study – Averting Thyroid Removal Surgery

Sandy, a 46-year-old woman, went to see my colleague, a Licensed Acupuncturist. A professional wedding singer, Sandy's singing ability deteriorated as her health declined, which forced her into early retirement. Around the same time, she was diagnosed with Hashimoto's thyroiditis and prescribed thyroid hormone therapy. She developed thyroid nodules and was informed by her medical doctor that she would need to have her thyroid removed. She wanted to keep her thyroid gland and sought out my colleague.

They worked together for three months with a diet that immediately eliminated all grains. Sandy increased her healthy protein intake with wild-caught fish, pasture-raised beef and free-range chicken. She also increased her fat consumption with avocados, raw butter, coconut oil and extra virgin, cold-pressed olive oil. Her daily consumption of cruciferous vegetables included broccoli, kale and Brussels sprouts. The acupuncturist also recommended kelp and other seaweeds. These foods, coupled with a three-week whole body detoxification program, shrunk all of her nodules, lowered her TPO auto-antibodies, and saved her thyroid. The following six months, the acupuncturist used specific whole food concentrates to regenerate her liver, adrenals, pituitary and thyroid glands. Her prescribing medical doctor gradually titrated her off her thyroid hormones when it was no longer required.

Through Sandy's committed work with my colleague, she became healthy and un-medicated. Her husband even noticed the greatest miracle of all — Sandy began singing again.

15

CROSSROADS

*"Two roads diverged in a wood, and I, I took the one
less traveled by, and that has made all the difference."*

— Robert Frost

We all make decisions – some poor, some good. Some bad decisions are based on incomplete or incorrect information. Even though the choice to work with a holistic health care practitioner is a road less traveled, it is a worthwhile one. Some courageous medical doctors have even ventured out to traverse the lands of the healing arts. They are holistic medical doctors who treat the cause of diseases instead of merely suppressing symptoms. They are the few, the strong, the brave – a minority.

Before the 1950s, most medical doctors were holistic. From the 1930-1950s, Dr. Royal Lee delivered lectures all over the country to medical doctors. Many of them even instructed their patients to consume whole food concentrates and observed countless healing miracles. Dr. Lee was knowledgeable about every aspect of human physiology, the science and study of the function of the body's systems, organs and cells. His knowledge of the effectiveness of whole food concentrates to support the healing process is why medical doctors sought him out.

In 1937, Dr. Lee invented the endocardiograph, a tool for graphing heart sounds. Previously, most nutrition-minded healthcare providers depended on the subjective stethoscope for a reading of the heart. Dr. Lee invented this tool to provide practitioners with an objective, accurate and detailed recording for evaluating the health of the heart and nutritional status.

For years, Dr. Lee traveled across the U.S. and taught chiropractors, cardiologists and other medical professionals how to use this device because it could detect nutritional deficiencies and imbalances long before a patient experienced symptoms. The endocardiograph amplifies and records both audible and inaudible heart sounds as the blood moves through the various chambers, valves and vessels over a five-minute period. This device demonstrated that the heart almost instantly reflects changes in body chemistry immediately after ingesting specific whole food concentrates.

The endocardiograph signature reflects the opening and closing of the valves, the contraction and strength of the heart muscles, and the efficiency of the movement of the blood, thus giving a clear view of heart function. It allows health care professionals to record the location, duration and intensity of murmurs and to hear variations too slight to be detected with a stethoscope.

In contrast, the modern electrocardiograph (EKG) used in hospitals today only records the surface electrical impulse as it moves through the nerves of heart tissue. The EKG primarily indicates if the heart's nervous tissue network has experienced trauma or permanent damage to its electrical functioning. Unfortunately, it will not discriminate valve function, muscle efficiency, nutritional deficiencies, etc.

Medical doctors and cardiologists who practiced medicine in the 1940s and 50s provided Dr. Lee's whole food concentrates to patients. Over time, they are becoming a rarity. Why are modern day medical doctors choosing not to incorporate whole food nutrition into their practice when it was used by the doctors before them with great success? A look into history shows us that many medical doctors took a detour down a slippery slope and never found their way back to the road of healing with whole food nutrition.

THE DOUBLE STANDARD OF CARE

As Dr. Lee lectured across the country to teach cardiologists about the endocardiograph, he also used it to demonstrate and record the efficacy of his whole food concentrates. He even compared the physiological improvements of these concentrates to those of the pharmaceutical chemicals at the time. One study done with a heart tissue extract showed that within fifteen minutes of taking it, a patient's electrocardiogram detected it and the electrical fields shifted to match a healthy person's. This clinical study, done in the 1940s, went on to show that this heart tissue extract proved more efficacious for patients with cardiovascular disease than the contemporary pharmaceutical. Unfortunately, at that moment the American Medical Association (AMA) and FDA began to redefine the scope of medicine in America to preserve the commercial interests of large pharmaceutical companies.

Today the Fortune 500 pharmaceutical companies are collectively referred to as "Big Pharma." If an allopathic medical doctor today wanted to become a holistic healer, they could implement whole food nutrition and begin to help their patients regenerate organs. However, it would require great sacrifice because the insurance companies, AMA, FDA and other organizations have developed a "standard of care," a medical or psychological treatment guideline that can be broad or narrow, specifying appropriate treatment based on scientific evidence of patented technologies or agents in the treatment of a given condition.

Even though Dr. Lee had collected evidence to support the efficacy of his whole food concentrates in restoring health to patients, foods are not patentable, so the "standard of care" no longer includes whole food nutrition. The road commonly traveled by allopathic doctors and patients is primarily focused on disease management or "sick care." Today's medical students receive a mere eight hours of formal nutritional training during medical school – sponsored by pharmaceutical companies, who spend these few hours declaring that nutritional therapy does not work and dictating pharmaceutical intervention for all patients with a diagnosable disease. The standard of care has significant gaps, which is why many allopathic doctors are incapable of successfully healing someone diagnosed with fibromyalgia or chronic fatigue syndrome. When the AMA prohibited licensed medical doctors from including whole food nutrition in their standard of care, they lowered the standard of health.

Though "Big Pharma" closed the curtains around Dr. Lee, his tissue extracts, whole food concentrates and the endocardiograph, a new era of light was born. Doctors of Chiropractic, Licensed Acupuncturists, Certified Nutritionists, Traditional Naturopaths, holistic Osteopaths, and holistic Medical Doctors are the new breed of holistic health care practitioners who carry the torch of whole food nutrition. They are waiting to support your healing body.

HEALTH INSURANCE

Many Americans inappropriately view health insurance as medical expense coverage. Insurance is a contract in which the insurer agrees to compensate the insured, or policyholder, for specified loss or damage from certain perils or risks in exchange for a fee, the insurance premium. For example, an automobile insurance company may agree to bear the risk that your car will be damaged in an automobile accident. According to the terms of your plan, they agree to help you repair your vehicle or replace it if it is deemed a total loss.

The creation of health insurance also had the same intention – covering damage, if necessary.

Before the development of health insurance, patients were expected to pay all other health care costs out of their own pockets – regular office visits, treatment and any medicine. Hospital surgeries, stays and other services were also paid out of pocket, also known as fee-for-service.

Health insurance was first offered in the United States by the Health Assurance Company in Massachusetts during the late 1800s. This firm sold insurance against injuries arising from railroad and steamboat accidents, which today is known as "catastrophic coverage" – severe and sudden trauma that requires expensive life saving hospital care.

During the middle of the 20th century, many more companies offered health insurance. Policies and programs have evolved and now cover routine doctor visits, emergency health care procedures and prescription drugs. They collect premiums from you and reimburse your doctor for any rendered services. Unfortunately, health insurance companies have turned into really wealthy middleman corporations. Their original role of providing catastrophic care to patients who run into unfortunate accidents has deceptively transformed into negotiating brokers who convince the public to pay high premiums, and partially reimburse medical professionals for rendered services.

Health insurance companies have created a financial black hole in an already broken healthcare system. As an example, a doctor provides $200 worth of services to a patient. The patient (and/or employer) pays the health insurance company a $200 monthly premium. The doctor receives $60 reimbursement leaving $140 for the health insurance company to cover labor costs for its staff and dividends to owners and investors.

Many health insurance providers convince the public to pay high monthly premiums and receive "sick care" in the form of pharmaceuticals, radiation and surgery. Not all health care plans allow a person to regularly see a holistic health care practitioner for whole food nutrition, acupuncture or chiropractic care, which address the cause of many health concerns.

The value of insurance is for emergency "what if" scenarios. I recommend always having health insurance to protect you and your family. Look for a low premium, high-deductible catastrophic coverage policy, so that you are covered if a traumatic accident requires immediate surgery or hospitalization. It is my sincerest hope that none of us will ever have to use it.

History has shown us many forks along the roads of life. Louis Lasagna removed the directive to use food as medicine from the Hippocratic Oath in 1964; the FDA forced Harvey Wiley, the last honest guardian of healthy foods from his government post in 1912; the AMA banned the use of Dr. Lee's whole food concentrates in the 1950s and forever altered the "standard of care" that allopathic medical doctors abide by. However, the power to improve our health and the health of our children depends on the decisions we make and the stand we take. Each of us is personally responsible for our own health, degeneration or regeneration. Every pharmaceutical corporation, food manufacturer, and health insurance broker, wants to collect our hard earned money. We ultimately vote with our hard earned dollars by how we choose to spend them.

Isn't it time for you to take the road less traveled?

Question #2 to ask yourself:
Do I have a catastrophic health insurance policy to provide coverage for emergency and hospital related services?

16

EAT TO THRIVE

"One of the biggest mistakes that medical science has ever made: to provide drugs to people who are starving. A starving man doesn't need drugs. He needs food. And if he gets food he recovers."

— Dr. Royal Lee

Belinda came into my office in May of 2010 for her very first nutritional evaluation. Like many of my nutrition clients, she believed my job as a nutritional consultant is to tell people to not eat another bite of their favorite foods. She admitted that her fear was that she would have to give up her life's greatest joys. She spent years accumulating an extensive list of her city's finest restaurants. It is a myth that the only good nutritional advice is to cease and desist eating any unhealthy food. That type of nutritional consulting is hardly effective and risks creating hungry clients who remain clueless about which of the foods they eat are actually healthy. Belinda believed she was going to starve, which created doubt about making lifestyle changes.

"Contrary to what you've heard, Belinda, my job is to tell you about all the delicious foods you should be eating. And to eat enough of them, so your body is no longer starving." She was there because of organ degeneration and intolerable symptoms. I examined her food log, paying attention to the healthy foods she was already eating. I found she consumed them in insufficient quantities. It's easy to increase consumption of foods we are already familiar with. With each consultation, Belinda understood more clearly which of the foods she already ate were the healthier choices.

Belinda enjoyed eating wild-caught salmon, pasture-raised beef and eggs from free-range chickens. Her first assignment was to include at least three eggs or three ounces of salmon or beef with every meal, especially breakfast.

Few of my clients actually consume sufficient amounts of the necessary building blocks the healing body needs, including complete proteins, healthy oils and essential fats.

THE BUILDING BLOCKS OF LIFE

The word "protein" is derived from a Greek root meaning "of first importance." Protein makes up roughly one-fifth of a person's total weight and is the basic material of life. Protein plays multiple roles in the human body and serves as building blocks for most bodily structures — bones, muscles, arteries and veins, hair, skin and fingernails. Our brain, heart, lungs, liver and kidneys are constructed of tissue made of various proteins. They help carry the oxygen that reddens our blood. Enzymes are proteins that digest our food, synthesize essential substances, and break down waste products for elimination. Protein is needed to transport fat, cholesterol and mineral nutrients throughout the body. It is required for the production of certain hormones made by the adrenal and thyroid glands. Protein is also an effective energy source.

Since protein is needed to build nearly every organ and tissue in the body, protein deficiency is a serious issue. In adults, strong bones are made up of collagen Type 1 protein. Collagen protein comprises a third of bone volume, but is responsible for 70% of bone strength. Being short on protein is to lack the very substance that provides structure. Growing children, especially, need large amounts of protein. If they do not get enough of the right kind, growth and development suffers. In the unborn child and young infant, too little protein can stunt a child's growth — and no amount of protein consumed later in life can repair that damage. Protein deficient infants may face a lifetime of being smaller, weaker and less vital than their peers.

Muscle tissue is damaged by strenuous exercise, but our body repairs the damaged tissue with protein. Proteins are constantly broken down and rebuilt — known as protein turnover. Proteins break down into peptides, which are chains of amino acids, the smallest building blocks of proteins. Our bodies need continual replacement through daily intake of high quality protein. This process begins at conception and lasts throughout life, so without sufficient dietary protein intake, growth and all bodily functions will not be optimal.

> **Food for Thought:** The body has the ability to convert 1 gram of protein into 4 calories of energy. For this conversion, the kidneys must remove nitrogen from the amino acids. This process is called deamonization. The allopathic medical community often warns against the consumption of protein in patients whose kidney function is declining. Most cases of kidney failure are due to the overconsumption of toxic chemicals (including pharmaceuticals) and cadmium toxicity. The kidneys partner with the liver and lymph tissues to detoxify pharmaceutical drugs. Over time, the kidneys become taxed and show extreme signs of deterioration. Eating protein rebuilds kidney tissue while many pharmaceuticals destroy it and even cause interstitial nephritis (inflammation in the kidneys). Protein is important for optimal health. Check with your holistic health care practitioner who understands the value of high quality protein to the healing body.

Nearly all foods in a raw and unrefined state contain protein. Certain foods are proportionately higher in protein than others. Beef, chicken and pork contain more grams of protein than the same serving volume of collard greens which contain more fiber and water.

Beef, chicken, pork and other flesh meats are 10-40% protein. Almonds and other nuts are roughly 25% protein, mixed in with fats, oils, fiber, minerals and other nutrients. The protein content of cooked grains, beans, lentils and peas ranges from 3 to 10 percent. Potatoes, fruits and leafy green vegetables have 3% protein or lower.

Animal Source	Protein (g)	Plant Source	Protein (g)
Chicken (3 oz.)	27	Tempeh (4 oz.)	17-21
Turkey (3 oz.)	25	Lentils (½ cup)	9
Beef, (3 oz.)	24	Sunflower Seeds (½ cup)	13
Pork (3 oz.)	25	Soybeans (½ cup)	11
Tuna (3 oz.)	26	Kidney beans (½ cup)	8
Yogurt (8 oz.)	12	Black beans (½ cup)	8
Milk (8 oz.)	8	Chick-peas (½ cup)	8
Cheese (1 oz.)	7	Hummus (¼ cup)	5
Cream Cheese (2 TBSP)	4	Pinto beans, cooked (½ cup)	7
Egg (1 medium)	6	Lima beans, cooked (½ cup)	5
Cottage Cheese (½ cup)	14	Almonds (½ cup)	15
Cod (3 oz.)	20	Pine Nuts (½ cup)	15
Salmon (3 oz.)	22	Cashews (½ cup)	10
Shrimp (3 oz.)	21	Walnuts (½ cup)	10
Lobster (3 oz.)	17	Flax Seeds, ground (2 TBSP)	4

The human body requires protein for many reasons, so it is important to consume sufficient amounts of high protein foods. A good rule of thumb is to consume 0.75 grams of protein for every pound of body weight; e.g., 120 grams for a 160-pound person. This amount of daily protein intake can aid in the prevention and even reversal of osteoporosis.[175] For athletes and active people who require additional tissue repair, protein intake should be increased.

These figures assume that you eat a mixed diet of proteins that match the amino acid ratios required by the body. There are twenty-two different amino acids that are important to the body. These combine together in thousands of intricate biochemical patterns to create a variety of complex protein structures. Nine of the amino acids are "essential" — the body cannot produce them so they must be supplied from whole food sources.[176]

Foods that supply a specific ratio of the nine essential amino acids are considered to contain "complete protein." Virtually all proteins from raw animal foods are complete. Foods that lack one or more of the essential amino acids, such as certain fruits, grains and vegetables, contain "incomplete protein." Plant foods can be excellent sources of protein if eaten in combinations that supply the balance of essential amino acids. For example, in Latin cultures, the incomplete amino acid profile of beans combined with incomplete whole grain rice creates a balanced complete amino acid profile.

Essential Amino Acids	Nonessential Amino Acids
Histadine	Alanine
Isoleucine	Arginine
Leucine	Asparagine
Lysine	Aspartic acid
Methionine	Cysteine
Phenylalanine	Glutamic acid
Threonine	Glutamine
Tryptophan	Glycine
Valine	Ornithine
	Proline
	Serine
	Taurine
	Tyrosine

When we eat whole foods, a healthy digestive system breaks proteins down into its amino acids that enter the body's "pool" of amino acids. Each cell assembles the proteins it needs using the amino acids as building blocks. If one or more of the "nonessential" amino acids is in short supply, the body can produce it from essential ones.

However, low consumption of any essential amino acid can limit the body's effective use of the others. The body then cannot form protein, and isolated amino acids begin to accumulate in the bloodstream. Missing one of the essential amino acids is like trying to build a car on an assembly line without the engine. Supplies of tires, chassis, seats, brakes and windows keep arriving, but no cars can be completely built. Meanwhile, inventory of all these parts creates congestion in the manufacturing plant.

We need the nine essential amino acids in our diet as raw materials in just the right proportions and at the same time. It does little good taking in a few essential amino acids one day and getting the others later in the week.

Cooking protein with high heat destroys enzymes and other proteins. Lysine, methionine, cysteine and tryptophan are heat-labile (meaning susceptible to alteration or destruction), so are rendered unusable. Since lysine and methionine are essential amino acids, they must be attained by the consumption of protein in a raw state.

If you eat every food cooked, baked, grilled, stir fried, deep fried, pasteurized, etc., your body will develop deficiencies in the heat-labile amino acids, creating an overflow inventory of others. The primitive peoples studied by Dr. Price consumed raw animal and vegetable protein. They consumed eggs, milk, cheese, beef, chicken, fish, germinated nuts, sprouted seeds, plants and vegetables often in a raw, uncooked or fermented state.

One example of a raw protein food is Pemmican. It is a highly nutritious, food that is traditionally prepared by the natives of North America.[177] It is a concentrated mixture of fat and raw protein, usually prepared with the raw meat of large game such as bison, elk or deer.[178] The meat is thinly cut and then dried in the sun until hard and brittle enough to crush into a powder. It is then mixed with melted animal fat in equal proportions. Pemmican can be kept for months when left dry and packed into specially made rawhide pouches for storage.

Today, many restaurants serve delicious and savory raw meat dishes that include raw fish (sashimi, tuna tartare, poke) and raw beef (beef carpaccio, steak tartare, yuk hwe, kibbeh nayeh, kitfo, mettwurst, teewurst, koi soi, gyu tataki, bo tai chanh, carne apace). *Primal Diet* by Aajonus Vonderplanitz provides numerous raw meat recipes. A few are provided in *Nourishing Traditions* by Sally Fallon. Raw plant based dishes include raw vegetables, fruits, nuts, seeds, seaweeds, spices and other herbs. *Rawvolution* by Cherie Soria is an excellent resource filled with wonderful raw vegetable and nut based recipes.

It is important to eat only 100% pasture raised, organically grown animals. If you do eat beef, chicken, lamb or pork as a source for raw complete protein, avoid animals raised on a factory farm under commercial methods because of the exposure to antibiotics, vaccines and growth hormones. Organic eggs should come from chickens that are given "free range" to run around hunting for moving objects. Organic eggs have never been reported to be contaminated with salmonella. Buy only fresh raw nuts from organic farmers. Nuts fresh in their shells are better than de-shelled ones that have aged in a bin or plastic container. Many nuts have had their nutrients destroyed or altered after being roasted, irradiated, toasted or left sitting on shelves for extended periods of time.

If you don't raise animals or grow your own vegetables, it may not always be safe to consume foods that are 100% raw. The primitive cultures always knew who raised their cattle and who farmed the land — often it was themselves. They did not outsource. They practiced natural and organic methods of animal husbandry and farming. Wild animals were sometimes caught and wild crafted herbs and vegetables were gathered. These were safe to consume because their landscapes were free from chemical pollution. To identify local producers of organically grown produce and pasture raised animals in your area, visit www.eatwild.com or www.localharvest.org.

THE FATS OF LIFE

Belinda's husband Bob came in to see me when he saw her health improve. He began increasing raw protein intake at breakfast and noticed an improvement in his energy levels, then he came in to see if nutritional deficiencies caused any of his other symptoms — aching knee joints, dry skin on his hands, chapped lips, peeling skin on his feet and awful sunburns every time he tended the garden.

> **Case Study – Overcoming Chronic Fatigue Syndrome**
>
> At 48, Belinda complained of low to no energy. She was diagnosed with Chronic Fatigue Syndrome (CFS) three years prior and experienced extreme bowel discomfort whenever she ate beef, pork, fish or chicken.
>
> Her nutritional evaluation revealed that her stomach produced insufficient hydrochloric acid (HCl), a component for thorough digestion of protein. She also showed signs of pancreatic insufficiency. These issues are commonly brought on by diets excessively low in trace minerals (such as zinc) and vitamins, among other nutrients.
>
> She implemented a specific regimen of whole food concentrate formulas to restore the health to the organs responsible for regulating digestion — stomach, spleen, pancreas, liver, gallbladder and parasympathetic autonomic nervous system — which enabled her to digest protein effectively. Her program included protein rich foods at every meal, including breakfast. Her energy became stable throughout the day and she even began to sleep better throughout the night. Belinda's medical doctor was impressed with her improvements, declared her diagnosis (of three years) was a mistake — she no longer presented signs or symptoms of CFS — and suggested continuation of whatever she was doing.

Already consuming protein, he next increased his intake of healthy fats and oils which lubricate the body. He was shocked at my suggestion. "But, I'm afraid I'll gain weight. My medical doctor says I should be mindful of my caloric intake."

I explained that counting calories has misguided the public to associate excessive weight gain with the consumption of high caloric foods and a lifestyle of minimal exercise. This belief does not discriminate between the different types of calories and the specific hormones they signal the body to release. Specific calories from digested foods influence the body's release of insulin, which signals the body to store excess energy in adipose tissue (as fat). Other types of calories instruct hormones like glucagon to burn energy from fat reserves. *Good Calories, Bad Calories* by Gary Taubes does a phenomenal job of dismantling the "calories in, calories out" myth. Not all calories are created equal.

There are many hormones involved with regulating weight gain and weight loss. The majority of them are controlled by food choices, exercise routine, sleep cycle, stress level and chemical toxins, including pharmaceuticals. All nature-made fats are healthy and necessary for our healing bodies. The fourteen primitive cultures studied by Dr. Price consumed calories from healthy fats and oils that represented 30-80% of their diets, yet they were free from all disease and physical degeneration.

Every oil or fat provided to us by nature from whole food sources, when left unrefined and unadulterated, helps our body in numerous ways. They provide a concentrated source of energy, as well as the building blocks for cell membranes and a variety of hormones and hormone-like substances. Fats carry important fat-soluble Vitamins A, D, E, F, K and other nutrients such as CoQ10. Dietary fats are needed for the conversion of carotenoids to the active forms of the Vitamin A complex and play a vital role in the health of bones and endocrine glands. Fats transport calcium and many trace minerals, such as iodine, to the various tissues of the body. Raw and unrefined fats (and oils) strengthen the immune system and decrease systemic inflammation.[179] This is observed when high sensitivity C-Reactive Protein (CRP), an indicator of systemic inflammation, is lowered by the consumption of foods high in fat, like tuna.[180] There is growing evidence that systemic inflammation is the major cause of heart disease. Lipoprotein (a), another substance in the blood that indicates systemic inflammation, lowers with increased saturated fat intake, which also fuels the heart muscle.[181,182] The heart draws on its reserve of fat as an energy source in times of stress. Fat is also the precursor material for a majority of hormones. Hormones are the body's messengers and are critical for the optimal functioning of our brain, digestive, nervous and reproductive systems. To not eat fat is to intentionally starve the endocrine system.

Food for Thought: Fatty acids are classified as saturated, polyunsaturated and monounsaturated. A saturated fatty acid contains a hydrogen atom at all available carbon bonds, which makes them highly stable. Your body makes saturated fatty acids and they are found higher in animal fats and tropical oils. Polyunsaturated fatty acids have two or more pairs of double bonds and, therefore, lack four or more hydrogen atoms. Polyunsaturated fatty acids include omega-6 and omega-3 fatty acids, the omega number indicating the position of the first double bond. Monounsaturated fatty acids like omega-9 and omega-7, lack two hydrogen atoms.

The polyunsaturated fatty acids, linoleic acid and alpha-linolenic acid, are considered essential fatty acids (EFA) because the body cannot produce them, so we must consume them from whole foods, like nuts, seeds and vegetables. Both of these must be converted in our bodies into longer chain fatty acids to serve a beneficial biological function. Alpha-linolenic acid converts into docosahexaenoic acid (DHA), eicosapentaenoic acid (EPA) and prostaglandin E3 (PG-E3). Between 50-60% of the dry weight of the adult brain is lipid, and $1/3$ of these lipids are mostly DHA.[183,184] Unfortunately, many of us are deficient in the nutrients and minerals required to convert linoleic and alpha-linolenic acids into the longer chain fatty acids. Tuna, krill, calamari, cod and many other fish and animals that eat alpha-linolenic acid containing foods will produce DHA, EPA and PG-E3. When we eat whole animal foods, we receive these longer chained polyunsaturated fatty acids and can benefit from them immediately, rather than rely on our own body's resources and enzymes to produce them. While linoleic and alpha-linolenic acid are considered essential, it is more suitable for people who are clinically undernourished to eat both animal and plant sourced fats and oils.

We should avoid food products that contain trans fatty acids, including shortening, hydrogenated oils, margarine and most phony

'butter' spreads. The falsehood that saturated fat in butter being bad
for us is based on a myth. Nearly all fats and oils exist as a
combination mixture of saturated fatty acids, polyunsaturated fatty
acids and monounsaturated fatty acids — regardless of animal or plant
origin. Unfortunately, the media has led the public to believe that fats
and oils exist singly as one type of fatty acid. This is not the case
when you look at raw fats and oils from unrefined whole food
sources. Olive oil contains 16% saturated fatty acids, 11%
polyunsaturated fatty acids, and 73% monounsaturated fatty acids.
Coconut oil, now touted as one of the greatest health foods, especially
helpful in the treatment of patients with Alzheimer's disease, is 91%
saturated fat and 7% monounsaturated.[185] See Figure 19. Public media
has again provided dietary misdirection by telling us to avoid
saturated fats. They are all important for the healing body to thrive.

The main differentiating factor between a fat and oil is the
temperature that it becomes a solid (fat) or a liquid (oil). Animal fats
such as butter, lard and tallow contain 40-60% saturated fat and are
solid at room temperature. Vegetable oils, such as olive and peanut oil
from northern climates, contain a majority of polyunsaturated fatty
acids and are liquid at room temperature. Vegetable oils from the
tropics, such as coconut and palm oil, are highly saturated.[†††] Coconut
oil is liquid in the warmer tropics, but hard as butter in cooler
locations. Plants must maintain additional stiffness in the hot climates
of the tropics, so they naturally produce an increased proportion of
saturated fatty acids.

The higher the saturated fat content of a fat or oil means it
becomes solid at a lower temperature. All fats will turn liquid as the
temperature rises. All oils turn solid as temperature drops. The
temperature at which this occurs depends on the ratio of saturated
fatty acids to unsaturated fatty acids.

The essential fatty acids go rancid (oxidize) quite easily,
particularly linoleic acid and alpha-linolenic acid, so must be treated
with care. Polyunsaturated oils oxidize when subjected to heat,
oxygen and moisture from cooking or processing. Rancid oils are

---

[†††]The production of commercial palm oil primarily requires destruction of rainforest, especially
remaining orangutan habitat in Borneo and Sumatra.

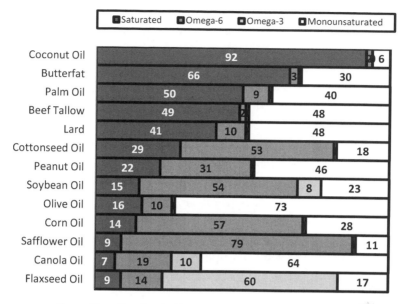

Source: Know Your Fats by Mary G. Enig, PhD

Figure 19. General composition of various oils and fats by percentage.

characterized by free radicals — single atoms or clusters with an unpaired electron in an outer orbit — that cause many health problems. They are associated with premature aging, autoimmune diseases such as arthritis, Parkinson's disease, Lou Gehrig's disease, Alzheimer's and cataracts. [186] With extreme chemical reactivity, they attack cell membranes and red blood cells, damage DNA/RNA strands and trigger mutations in tissue, blood vessels and skin. Free radical damage to the skin causes wrinkles and premature aging, where as free radical damage to tissues and organs sets the stage for tumors. Since most fats and oils contain polyunsaturated oils, they should never be heated or used in cooking. Commercially sold oils that are high in rancid polyunsaturated fatty acids include the common vegetable oils.

Avoid these oils, as most of them are highly processed:

- Canola Oil
- Soybean Oil
- Corn Oil
- Safflower Oil
- Cottonseed Oil
- Grapeseed Oil
- Sunflower Oil

Organic, extra-virgin and cold-pressed olive oil is safe to consume, for it has not been exposed to the harsh conditions of refining. The term "extra-virgin" indicates it is unrefined and "cold-pressed" indicates heat was not used during the extraction process. Choose those that are packaged in dark bottles, since exposure to sunlight can cause the polyunsaturated fatty acids portion of olive oil to oxidize.

When selecting oils for cooking, select those with a higher proportion of saturated fatty acids, which are stable at higher temperatures and will not go rancid as easily as polyunsaturated fatty acids. Coconut oil, butter, ghee, tallow and lard are preferred choices for cooking because of their high saturated fatty acid content. Always choose raw and organic versions of these oils.

Avoid heating fats and oils whenever possible, since raw fats and oils contain many nutrients that are heat-labile. The fats found in raw soybeans, raw cream and raw butter contain nutrients — such as the Wulzen or "anti-stiffness" factor — that help lubricate the joints and support liver function. These nutrients protect against calcification of the joints, essentially preventing degenerative joint conditions such as arthritis. They also protect the arteries, eyes and pineal gland, lubricates joints, skin, eyes and areas of muscle aches and cramps.[187] These benefits are destroyed by pasteurization (over heating) and homogenization (excess blending) of milk.

All cell membranes are made out of phospholipid bilayers (lipid means fatty acid) mainly made from long chain polyunsaturated and saturated fatty acids that give cells flexibility and integrity. Healthy cell membranes also contain cholesterol which adds stiffness and stability. When a person takes a cholesterol-lowering drug, such as a statin, and consumes a low fat diet, their dividing cells have difficulty producing new membranes due to insufficient raw materials. These malformed cells steal from tissues rich in fat and oil composition — nerve tissue and the brain. Nerve pain, brain fog or inability to focus can be signs that healthy fat intake from raw whole food sources is inadequate.

If trans fats and rancid oils replace healthy fats and oils in our body, cell membranes become fragile with pores and breaks that allow substances — including toxins and viral vectors — to enter, which

Food for Thought:

Nature does not make bad fats. Humans take good fats and convert them into something dangerous to our health. Most vegetables oils have undergone a gruesome refining process. Canola oil, soy oil, sunflower oil, cottonseed oil, corn oil, grape seed oil, safflower oil, margarine and non-butter spreads typically have been highly refined. Canola oil is removed by a combination of high temperature mechanical pressing and toxic solvent extraction. Traces of the solvent (almost always hexane) remain in the oil, despite attempts to remove it via caustic refining, bleaching and degumming (which involves high temperatures or chemicals that are not always safe for human consumption.) Since canola oil is high in polyunsaturated fatty acids, it becomes rancid and foul smelling from the process. Thus, it must be deodorized by a process that converts a large portion of the fatty acids into *trans* (or hydrogenated) fatty acids.

The University of Florida at Gainesville's research on commercial vegetable oils found the *trans* fat levels to be as high as 4.6%.[188] Unfortunately, this is not on the labels, so consumers are unaware of what is actually in the bottle. Hydrogenated canola oil can be found in many processed foods because higher levels of *trans* fatty acids confer longer shelf life, a crisper texture in cookies and crackers and ultimately more profits for junk food manufacturers — as well as elevated rates of chronic disease for the consumer.[189]

further weakens the cell. A weakened cell membrane will also leak contents from the cytoplasm out of the cell and into the blood. The immune system, responsible for detecting and identifying foreign particles in the blood, including these intracellular components, develops antibodies to these "foreign" substances. The first layer of preventing any autoimmune condition from escalating is to restore the strength of cellular membranes with healthy lipids and cholesterol. A complete halt to the consumption of any food containing rancid oils or trans-fatty acids is a must for the health of every cell.

There are fatty acids throughout every living cell of our bodies. The average woman is made up of 25-31% fat, while the average man 18-24%.[190] The primitive cultures that Dr. Price studied were healthy because they consumed a variety of raw, fermented and some cooked fats with no damage to their health. Most people, especially infants and growing children, benefit from *more* fat in the diet rather than less. But the fats we eat must be chosen with care.

Avoid all processed foods containing dehydrogenated or hydrogenated fats and oils. Instead, use fats from pork (lard), cow (tallow), duck, goose and chicken; coconut oil, butter, ghee, traditional vegetable oils like extra virgin olive oil, and small amounts of unrefined flax seed oil; and only in organic, cold-pressed or raw forms. Butter and ghee should be raw from cows that are pasture raised. Organic butter, extra virgin olive oil and raw coconut oil are available in most health food stores and gourmet markets. Avocados, nuts (including walnuts, almonds, pecans, cashews, peanuts) and seeds (including sunflower, pumpkin, sesame) can also be an excellent source of fats and oils. Be sure they are always organic, fresh and unrefined.

CARBOHOLICS ANONYMOUS

In October of 1933, Dr. Royal Lee stated: "Candy, all white sugar or its products, and white flour including its products such as macaroni, spaghetti, crackers, etc., should be absolutely barred from the diet of the child. All these are energy-producing foods that do not contain any building materials for the body. The consequences of their toleration are susceptibility to infections, enlarged tonsils, carious teeth, unruly dispositions, stunted growth, rickets, poor development and very often permanent damage to many organs of the body (especially the endocrine glands) that depend upon the vitamin supply for their normal function and development." In 1942, the American Medical Association issued this public statement: "The consumption of sugar and of other relatively pure carbohydrates has

> **Case Study - Rheumatoid Arthritis**
>
> Bob had challenges digesting fatty foods. He was also diagnosed with rheumatoid arthritis and was taking anti-inflammatory and immunosuppressant medications. From his nutritional evaluation, it was clear he required immediate help to restore function to most of his fat digesting organs — salivary glands, liver, gallbladder, spleen and pancreas. We spent two months restoring his fat digestion capability, while providing his body with healthy fats and oils from raw organic coconut oil, olive oil, raw butter and avocados. With a specific regimen of whole food concentrate formulas, health was restored to the organs responsible for fat digestion and immunity, including bone marrow, spleen, thymus and liver. We strengthened his innate immune system while calming his immune reaction, which lowered his auto-antibody count without increasing risk of infection.
>
> After eleven months, his medical doctor declared he no longer had rheumatoid arthritis and removed all medications. Bob's medical doctor was impressed with his improvements and suggested continuation of what he was doing. By Bob eating protein and raw fats at every meal, he remains healthy and un-medicated.

become so great during recent years that it presents a serious obstacle to the improved nutrition of the general public."[191] Sixty years later, one would expect the FDA, USDA or AMA to put warning labels on all foods that contain white sugar or white flour.

Nearly all prepared or packaged desserts contain sugar in some form, often sourced from sugar cane. It is a highly refined, isolated and crystallized substance. Because of its highly addictive nature, it should be considered the most dangerous substance on the planet. Refined sugars deplete the B complex vitamin stores in the body. In order to metabolize sugar and other refined carbohydrates for energy (in the form of adenosine triphosphate) through aerobic cellular respiration (the Krebs or TCA cycle), the body requires B complex vitamins and amino acids. Unfortunately, when their reserves of these nutrients are depleted, the muscles generate energy via anaerobic respiration processes that lead to muscle soreness.

Many people diagnosed with fibromyalgia and chronic fatigue syndrome are severely depleted in B complex vitamins, heat-labile amino acids, essential fatty acids and trace minerals. Their muscles are constantly utilizing anaerobic respiration, resulting in a buildup of lactic acid and other by-products that result in muscular soreness. The B complex vitamins are found highest in raw liver, nutritional yeast, the germ and bran portions of uncooked and sprouted grains. Liver is the optimal source of all three because it contains the active form of the B complex vitamins while the other sources contain precursors that must be converted to the active form by the body. High dosages of synthetic B vitamins, produced in laboratories from coal tar, will exacerbate an already existing B complex deficiency.

Many people equate refined carbohydrates to sugar. These are typically sourced from grains (wheat, corn, rice, etc.) with most of their nutrients (essential fatty acids, B complex vitamins, trace minerals) removed by machinery for finer texture and prolonged shelf life. Complex carbohydrates (polysaccharides) eventually break down into simple sugars known as monosaccharides and disaccharides. These break down into glucose which enters cells with the hormone insulin. Cells typically do not require that much glucose, so extra glucose is converted into adipose tissue for storage. The overconsumption of sugar is a major contributor to the obesity epidemic. Glucose in the blood stream can also form advanced glycated end products (AGE's) and pentosidines, which are residues that may present as dark spots on the skin. These spots can eventually disappear by avoiding sugar, starches and carbohydrates and providing sufficient liver support. There are no *essential* sugars required in our diet to live optimally.

The evolutionary development of amylase, the enzyme our salivary glands secrete to digest starch, is thought to have enabled us to digest starches and complex carbohydrates. Fats and proteins can also be converted into glucose by a slow process that permits energy to be released over time. Humans have traditionally had more difficulty finding foods that contained substances quickly convertible into glucose. Hence, many of our hormones raise glucose levels and only one lowers it. See Figure 20.

Hormone	Tissue of Origin	Effects on Blood Glucose
Insulin	Pancreatic β-Cells	Lowers
Somatostatin	Pancreatic D Cells	Raises
Glucagon	Pancreatic α-Cells	Raises
Epinephrine	Adrenal Medulla	Raises
Cortisol	Adrenal Cortex	Raises
ACTH	Anterior Pituitary	Raises
Growth Hormone	Anterior Pituitary	Raises
Thyroxine	Thyroid	Raises

Figure 20. Hormones that raise or lower blood glucose.

Raw milk, whole grains, organic vegetables, fruits and root vegetables are healthy sources of carbohydrates. The Melvin Page Food Plan (in Chapter 10) categorizes vegetables according to carbohydrate percentages and places emphasis on vegetables that contain fewer carbohydrates so they can be consumed in unlimited amounts. These carbohydrate-containing foods also contain many nutrients that contribute to our health, but are lost when grains are refined to produce white flour and pure starches.

Question #3 to ask yourself:
Am I ready to upgrade my diet to ensure my body has the raw building blocks to repair itself?

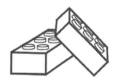

WATER - THE OTHER ESSENTIAL SUBSTANCE

Water makes up 60-70% of the human body. If we do not drink water for three days, our organs reach a state of shock and shut down. It is the medium that transports nutrients to our organs and tissues, while transporting toxins to our detoxification organs for excretion.

Water allows us to raise vegetables, fruit trees and animals. The Earth's surface is 70% water. It is essential to all species on the planet. Sadly, both bottled and municipal water are now contaminated with pharmaceutical drugs and other endocrine disrupting compounds.[192,193,194]

The best water is provided by nature from clean sources. I recommend seeking out a spring on www.findaspring.com. Health conscious citizens in your community provide the locations of spring water sources throughout the entire United States. Many of them have information on the safety of the water and their mineral contents. It is best to transport and store all raw and unrefined spring water in glass containers. Containers made from plastic carries the potential for it to leach into the water, which is not always safe for humans to consume. Bisphenol-A (BPA), a common substance in plastic bottles, has been shown to cause miscarriages, obesity, diabetes, insulin resistance and many other health challenges.[195,196,197] Many new plastic containers are BPA free, but there are many other substances in plastic that have not been studied and may have the same harmful effects.

When hydrating the healing body, a great rule of thumb is to consume half your body weight in ounces per day. A 100 pound person should drink 50 ounces each day. The best sources for water are spring water, raw milk (goat and cow), kefir, vegetables, fruits and homemade probiotic sodas.

DON'T OVERCOOK, FERMENT

It is better to consume foods with fewer steps of processing. With just one process, like charcoal grilling, we can convert a perfectly healthy steak from a 100% grass finished pasture raised cow into a heap of carcinogens by charbroiling it until it is black. Heterocyclic amines (HCAs) and polycyclic aromatic hydrocarbons (PAHs) form when muscle meat of beef, pork, fish or poultry is cooked at high-temperature, whether pan frying or grilling directly over an open flame.[198] These substances are carcinogenic and should always be avoided.

Cooking with heat sterilizes meats, breaks down indigestible fibers, and even helps release various nutrients. Many herbalists will boil herbs to extract the healing constituents. To make tea, an herbalist boils water to seep the beneficial elements from the leaf. Unfortunately, the mass media has made us fear bacterial infestations, so we tend to overheat and overcook nearly all of our food.

By going to such an extreme, we have destroyed a lot of nutrients, vitamins and proteins (including enzymes) that are essential to optimal health. When spinach is overcooked, it loses its bright green color and turns pale forest green. The color change indicates that the wonderful chlorophyll molecules that provide blood-building nutrients have lost their effective magnesium centerpiece.

Consuming foods raw or fermented is highly recommended. Prior to the widespread manufacturing of refrigerators in the 1940s, nearly everybody fermented or pickled vegetables and meats as a method of preserving. Cultures all over the world ferment grapes for wine and dairy for kefir, whey and cheese. Soybeans were fermented for tempeh and miso, bok choy for kimchi, cabbage for sauerkraut, wheat for beer or sourdough. In the south, Polynesians ferment taro for poi. In the north, Eskimos ferment meats, cod liver, and fish to produce "high meat". The Swedish ferment Baltic herring to make "Surströmming". The Koreans ferment skate, a cartilaginous fish, for "Hongeohoe" and the Japanese ferment mackerel and exocoetidae, also known as flying fish, to produce the odorous dish called "Kusaya".

The process of fermentation allows strains of beneficial bacteria that are probiotic (*pro* means "for" and *biotic* means "life") to thrive in our foods. Besides being an excellent method of preserving foods, fermentation replenishes the healthy bacteria (gut flora) in our digestive tracts. Vegetable-based ferments are mainly anaerobic lacto-fermented while high meats are primarily aerobically fermented, so the presence of a constant oxygen supply is integral.

Scientists have found that bacterial cells in the human body outnumber human cells ten to one. Commonly researched strains of beneficial bacteria include Lactobacillus acidophilus, Bifidobacterium longum, Lactobacillus paracasei and Saccharomyces cerevisiae boulardii. The mixed community of these bacterial cells does not threaten us but instead offers vital help with basic physiological processes, including immune self-defense. For example Saccharomyces boulardii is effective in preventing and treating patients who have develop diarrhea and colitis due to antibiotic resistant Clostridium difficile.[199,200]

In addition to fighting antibiotic induced infections, these beneficial bacteria help digest foods during the fermentation process, then release those nutrients that we ourselves cannot manufacture directly from the foods. They support the further breakdown of foods, enhance the body's ability to absorb essential dietary minerals, help produce specific nutrients (such as Vitamin K), and improve the absorption of water and lipids in the gastrointestinal tract.[201, 202] Fermentation enables preparation and storage of foods to retain and, in many cases, augment nutritional value. I recommend *Wild Fermentation* by Sandor Katz as your first guide in learning how to ferment. You will have a lifetime of recipes to explore in just that one book alone.

Food for Thought: If you consume a vegetarian diet (as I experimented with years ago) or plan on doing so, practice it safely. On occasion I will only consume vegetables for certain periods of times. Although no thriving culture has existed to successfully give birth to generations of healthy offspring on a vegan or vegetarian diet, the value of consuming vegetables to support specific organ function is priceless, especially since we live in a toxic environment polluted with unprecedented amounts of chemical toxins. Organic, especially the cruciferous, vegetables provide substantial amounts of phytonutrients to support the ability of our liver and kidneys to metabolize and excrete toxins from our body. *Primal Body-Primal Mind* by Nora Gedgaudas and *The Vegetarian Myth* by Lierre Keith are excellent reads to thoroughly understand the long-term risks and precautions of a vegetarian lifestyle.

17

PURIFICATION

"You are what you eat, absorb, assimilate,
metabolize and don't excrete."

— Anonymous

Beautiful Margot was 24 when she came into my office disappointed in her inability to lose excess weight after trying numerous diets. From her waist up, she fit the profile of a normal weight 5' 6" woman. However, from the waist down, it was a different story. It was as if her lower body belonged to another person. Her hips, thighs and buttocks were extremely swollen, turning her body into a pear shape. I suspected hormone replacement therapy — that included estrogen. I found that she had taken birth control pills for eight years. She attributed to the pill her weight gain and, in addition, an ill-temper. In particular, the latter had not been conducive to work efficiency among her employees at the candle factory she runs. Managing 80 manual laborers was not easy.

I scanned Margot's intake form for information about her bowel movements. She had left that section blank. "How many bowel movements did you have last week?"

"I had one bowel movement last week. That's usually my normal." I have observed that women with a long history of birth control usually develop constipation.

Poor Margot was misinformed that one bowel movement a week was normal. Her flaring temper is characteristic of the body's physical tension building up. Constipation means her body was unable to release toxins and waste. Severe constipation can turn heaven's angels into irritable demons nobody wishes to be around. No wonder her employees were always on edge around her.

Margot shared that she used the occasional laxative. However, when she used them too often, her body developed a tolerance and they were no longer effective. Regular bowel movements are very important and one of the easier issues to resolve. I assured her that elimination of toxins would normalize her weight. These stored agents were internally polluting her body. There is a saying, "The body's solution to pollution is dilution." Margot's body was retaining water systemically as a defense mechanism.

Constipation is a symptom of poor elimination health, like a clogged toilet that will never flush. These residues stick to the colon and lymph tissues. If the constipation can be relieved, unwanted waste will be freely flushed down the toilet. Detoxification of any birth control pill residues and other toxins would come next. Margot, like many other clients, was not quite ready to hear that FDA approved drugs need to be detoxified from the body.

DETOXIFICATION IS FOR EVERYONE

All humans undergo detoxification. Two main endotoxins (toxins produced by the body) are expected to be in our bloodstream, carbon dioxide (CO_2), which is a by-product of cellular respiration, and ammonia, a waste product from protein utilization. The blood transports CO_2 to the lungs where it is removed with every breath. The liver converts ammonia to urea which is excreted via the urine by the kidneys. Many of our organs are helping us detoxify constantly. Our livers, lungs and kidneys were designed to handle these toxins.

However, we live in a world today that increases our toxic load multi-fold. Our air, water and food contain toxins that affect our health and the health of all living things. In 2010, over three billion pounds of toxic chemicals were either dumped into public sewage or released into the ground, surface waters or air. [203] Environmental pollutants, pesticides and chemicals are in nearly every commercial product. Many processed foods contain chemical additives that are also toxic to our bodies.

The accumulation of chemicals fatigue and eventually exhaust our detoxification organs — the liver, kidneys, lymph, skin, lungs and bowels. Our organs are designed to rid the body from endotoxins, not environmental toxins, and so they are overburdened. The liver and kidneys conduct most of the detoxification through a two-step enzymatic process that neutralizes unwanted chemical compounds, converting a toxic chemical into a less harmful water-soluble substance. If the liver and kidneys become fatigued or clogged, the lymph and skin become secondary routes of excretion. This explains why some people develop skin disorders or stagnant lymph drainage. For example, painful breasts may indicate that lymph tissue near the mammary glands has drainage challenges. Stagnant lymph tissue in other areas can lead to pain of the low back, knees, groin, armpits, tonsils, etc. Supporting each of the detoxification pathways must always be a priority if you live in a toxic environment.

The liver has 2 main detoxification pathways: Phase I and Phase II. In Phase I, toxins are attached to a carrier molecule, similar to placing garbage into a bag. Phase II transports the toxins out of the body, similar to carrying trash out of the house. Both Phase I and Phase II pathways require sufficient nutrients that can only be found in foods. Vegetables, such as Brussels sprouts, kale, broccoli, buckwheat leaf, barley grass and alfalfa, contain compounds (glucosinolates, sulforaphane, sinigrin isothiocyanates, chlorophyll, bioflavanoids, etc.) which fuel and support the detoxification organs. Cruciferous vegetables are particularly high in nutrients such as indole-3-carbinols, which are shown to support the liver's ability to detoxify the body of chemicals, heavy metals and other toxins.[204,205,206,207,208] Beet root, chard, radish, cauliflower, milk thistle,

> **Food for Thought:** The detoxification pathways of Phase I and Phase II require the cytochrome P450 liver enzymes to metabolize toxins and render them water-soluble so they can be excreted out of the body via the urine, bile or sweat. The cytochrome P450 enzymes are also responsible for clearing and detoxifying most pharmaceutical drugs from the body.
>
> Caffeine and many other substances are made water-soluble and excreted by the kidneys. Caffeine is a diuretic because it increases activation of the Phase I detoxification pathway, preventing caffeine from remaining in the blood stream long-term.[209]

cilantro, garlic, hawthorn flower, red clover, burdock root, cayenne pepper, juniper berry and many other vegetables provide nutrients to support detoxification by the liver and entire healing body.

In addition to specific plants and botanicals, a raw complete protein source with a balanced amino acid profile is essential for liver Phase II amino acid conjugation. A complete purification program does not require anybody to starve or go hungry. Fasting is not always the best solution for detoxification. We should not abstain from consuming essential amino acids and other nutrients for too long.

Our liver and other detoxification organs were never intended to be exposed to the myriad of toxic chemicals we see today. The modern world is different from the days Dr. Price traveled the globe. The land, air and water of the fourteen villages he studied were much cleaner and contained significantly fewer environmental toxins, if any.

Since many environmental toxins enter our bodies as we breathe, eat or drink, our detoxification organs must receive additional nutrients just to manage the increased burden. Many of today's modern health issues are a result of the combination of malnutrition and extreme chemical toxicity. It is critical that we consume foods that are more nutrient dense than those our ancestors consumed. The fact that much of the food grown today contains fewer nutrients due to poor soil health and sub-par farming methods, compounds the need for supplementary nutrients to fuel detoxification pathways and address contemporary toxicity problems.

Organic whole food-based concentrates can provide a solution to the challenge of replenishing nutrient deficits to fuel all of the healing body's detoxification organs. Purification programs enhance the body's capacities to remove toxic by-products from normal metabolism and the toxic chemicals introduced from the environment.

WARNING: WEIGHT LOSS OCCURS IF OVERWEIGHT

Toxic substances such as heavy metals, chemicals or drugs that are not effectively removed become sequestered and stored into various tissues and organs — including adipose tissue, which is considered both a tissue and an organ.[210] The body's fat tissues store toxins if the body's detoxification organs are incapable of thoroughly removing them from the blood stream. Undergoing a purification program may reduce fat stores as the body releases fat-soluble toxins stored in adipose tissue.[211]

The opposite is also true. Underweight people may begin to build body mass. Weight is merely a phenotype (genetically expressed trait) of lifestyle, which includes dietary choices. Most people will also lose weight by eating nothing for three weeks or using illicit drugs that increase metabolism, but this does not represent vibrant health. Certain pharmaceutical medications alter metabolism, which causes weight gain or prevents the release of toxins from fat tissue. Weight should only be used as one indicator to measure changes from your lifestyle, not a reliable barometer of overall health.

MAKING THE LEAP

Prior to undergoing any purification program, make sure your digestion and bowel movements are healthy. Purification programs are designed to draw toxins out from storage in organs and tissues, route them from the bloodstream to the detoxification organs, and support elimination. Women who are pregnant or nursing can undergo a purification program, but they are highly encouraged to seek the guidance of a holistic health care practitioner who can reduce and eliminate the risk of transferring toxins to an unborn or nursing child.

Traditional Chinese Medicine practitioners apply cupping, which involves a pump or fire to remove oxygen from a cup to create a vacuum over areas of stagnant tissue. Coffee enemas are also helpful in supporting the liver, clearing the lymph and dilating the hepatic portal vein. An excellent resource to understand purification and other cleansing techniques are detailed in *Clinical Purification: A Complete Treatment and Reference Manual* by Gina Nick.

The process of purification is not just a physical experience. Many people may undergo an emotional detoxification when they give up addictive junk foods. In 2008, the average American consumed over 130 pounds of sugar a year.[212] During a purification program, withdrawal symptoms of sugar cravings can uncontrollably arise. Persevering through the purges of the urges requires discipline and will power. Acupuncture, acupressure, chiropractic and specific herbs are also known to support the removal of cravings for processed food or sugar. While purification is often a smooth process, there may be a pothole or two along the road to wellness.

When I was nine, I embarked the spinning teacups ride at Disneyland after eating three corndogs and two cinnamon buns. It was exhilarating. The world was a blur and I felt like I was flying among clouds. I briefly wondered when the ride would stop because I began to feel dizzy. When it finally ended, I stumbled out of the gates and found my family. I bent over and hurled the contents from my stomach onto some poor bystander's shoes. I felt immediately better, clearheaded and ready for the next ride. If you feel queasiness or discomfort during a purification program, know that it is temporary. Once the chemical toxins have been removed, you will feel more vibrant, energetic and healthy than you have in a long time.

Question #4 to ask yourself:
Am I ready to enhance the removal of toxins from my body with the support of a purification program?

Food for Thought: Corndogs contain sodium nitrates, which transforms into nitrosamine, a reactive compound that has been shown to promote cancer.[213] Cinnamon buns and other bread products often contain potassium bromate, also known to cause cancer.[214] Perhaps vomiting up these processed foods after a turbulent roller coaster ride is a blessing in disguise.

18

GENETICS ARE NOT YOUR DESTINY

"The first wealth is health."

— Ralph Waldo Emerson

Even by the most conservative geneticists' standards, we have anywhere from 80% to 97% control over the expression of our genes. We have dormant genes for all sorts of things, both good and bad. A person is not just overweight because their mother and father were overweight. One is not destined to have a heart attack just because half the people in their family have had one; nor by the same token, diabetes or cancer.

Genetics can have some influence, but genes are turned on and off by regulatory genes that are mainly controlled by nutrients. A gene will not express itself unless the internal environment is conducive to its expression. So we have control over our genetic expression by the foods we choose to eat, the emotions we habitually experience, and the thoughts we consciously allow to govern our minds. We choose our lifestyle and that, in turn, impacts the expression of our genes.

We can also deliberately address the toxicity of our body's internal environment. We all inherit our genetic code from our parents. While many physical features are genetically predetermined, they do little to define our health. The bad habits which we inherit impact us far more than we are willing to admit.

Learn to be the master of your own genetic destiny with the decisions you make each moment.

UPGRADING YOUR BODY

Many animals shed their fur (or molt) by completely losing their external skeleton to live a new life with a refreshed set of cells. My young niece was recently excited to share her science class project. She carried in a large glass aquarium, with multiple cocoons hanging inside. I was excited about her joy in biology and the continuous change that occurs in nature. She shared with me that in two weeks, their transformation into beautiful monarch butterflies would be complete.

We humans are the same. The healing body you have today is not the same one you had seven years ago. All cells replicate, die and are either removed from the body or dismantled into spare parts. For every cell that replicates, a newer one is born. This new cell has the potential to be stronger and healthier than its older twin, which will one day undergo apoptosis, an intrinsically timed cell death. In another few years, every cell, tissue and organ will belong to a completely new version of you.

Every cell in our body along with its components is totally replaced within nine months. Some cells have a faster turnover rate than others, but ALL cells are rejuvenated and replaced, even in our organs and endocrine glands. In the developing field of epigenetics, the biology of belief and behavior, we are learning more about how we live through our cells and can reach the full expression of our genetic potential. This becomes especially true when we live as our ancestors did in the hunter-gatherer days.

The empirical findings and nutritional tools put together by the pioneers of nutrition — Doctors Royal Lee, Melvin Page, Weston Price, Francis Pottenger and Harvey Wiley — have been offered for humanity to thrive. But in order to do so, we must eat better.

The foods we eat must be whole, fresh and unprocessed. To continue with a life of poor dietary habits and increased chemical consumption will inevitably lead to decreased vitality and unhealthy children; in short, the degeneration of the human race. We evolved eating certain foods in certain ways. No caveman has ever been known to trim the fat off of his meat — he ate the entire animal. No Alpine villager ate low fat cheese. The Maori fishermen never avoided shellfish for fear of cholesterol. They ate the cholesterol with all the fat. Real and whole foods are packaged how nature intended — containing all the nutrients for optimal assimilation by our bodies. Eating whole foods insures us of the highest value of nutrients our food has to offer. Tampering with them is ill advised.

CHEERS TO YOUR HEALTH

Life does not have to end the sad way that society, pharmaceutical companies and allopathic medical doctors want us to believe. Life ends when our mission is complete. Life is beautiful and will include years of accumulated wisdom for you to pass onto grandchildren and great-grandchildren. During the later years of our lives, mental acuity can become sharper, the body can remain mobile and our joy can be uncontainable.

We ALL can heal, regenerate and live in wellness. It may appear that you are regaining your youth in the process — do not be alarmed, but embrace the change. The five most important factors for achieving optimum health and vitality or reversing illness and disease are interdependent:

1) **Finding a holistic health care practitioner:** The word 'Doctor' means 'Teacher.' They will be able to guide you to positive lifestyle improvements; a healthy diet is among them. Learn from them as much as you can. Attend their monthly patient lectures.

2) **Equitable Exchange:** It costs money to be healthy; it costs more to be sick. The healer you eventually work with has invested time and tuition fees to learn their trade for your

benefit. They are often very affordable and will never turn a patient away due to financial constraints. Your life is worth multiples more than the amount you eventually pay them. If you grow vegetables in your organic garden, many will exchange the vegetables of your labor for their services.

3) **Initializing Effort:** Undergo a purification program, eat organic and whole foods, exercise, mend relationships and, above all else, enjoy every moment. You must do your part.

4) **Allowing Time:** Holistic healers are quite capable of undoing one year of degeneration with one month of serious healing work. Be patient and open to the experience.

5) **Brightening Attitude:** Above all, you must believe you can heal. Attitude is everything. Fill places of fear with courage. This is the most important factor of all.

Question #5 to ask yourself:
Am I ready to support my healing body?

CLOSING WORDS

The innocent children of the world should never lose a loving parent from avoidable illness. No hopeful person, adult or child, should be told they have an incurable disease. As Dr. Price confirmed, all disease and physical degeneration result from malnutrition. We must return to the roots of human health. Conversely, pharmaceutical medications and processed foods create an even more nutritionally impoverished and toxic population, leading to increased sickness and poorer health.

We really are ancient bodies living in a modern world. Society has ignored this concept for a very long time as every commercial advertisement fervently attempts to distract you with the lure of their "new and improved" industrial by-products and processed foods. These may leave you older and sicker, while real whole foods will always be the greatest technology of life, brought to you by the impeccable generosity of nature. Humans have done little to improve upon nature's gifts. They have created pesticides to enable conventional farmers to grow abounding volumes of food to ship to other nations. However, the pesticides now pollute our drinking water and food supply, and other nations are still starving. The true worth of "new and improved" means an increase in your quality of vibrant life and not just in the quantity of manufactured foodstuffs.

Human beings are a part of this earth. We are programmed to thrive on what the earth provides for our bodies. We must discriminate between what is provided by nature versus man-made analogs falsely presented as identical to their real counterparts. The artificial creates increased toxicity and leads to health problems. To learn about it now is better than to never have learned it at all.

My permaculture teacher, Paul Wheaton, always reminds me that we, together, can create a better world through learning the "good things, rather than being angry at the bad guys." It is time we listen intently to Mother Nature and pay close attention to how we were intended to live. Find a quiet spot at a local or national park — then sit and just listen. You will be amazed at all the things you can hear, smell, feel and see. As a deer walks by in the distance you may be able to hear and feel its breath or step, each of which creates an impression on the environment. As a pebble falling into a pond creates a ripple that meets another ripple triggered by a fish jumping to catch an insect, they merge in confluence to create a new ripple. These intersecting patterns are always present in motion. We can hear them if we're listening, see them when we're watching, and feel them as long as we're still breathing.

As you make a conscious decision to meditate, go for a hike, or grow organic vegetables in your backyard, you set a new ripple moving into the world. When you share the harvest from your garden with a neighbor, you strengthen that ripple, allowing it to travel further, longer. Learning and living well are contagious. All our actions are like pebbles creating ripples that constantly meet, blend and merge. By teaching your family and friends, no one knows where your influence stops. It never actually does.

Bring back the natural methods of homesteading, permaculture and biodynamic farming into your community. They are the technologies that work with the environment and will help to restore it. Connect with your local farmers. Locate a CSA and farmers market near you. Cultivate the herbalist in you by preparing a cup of tea from whole leaves. Learn about the healing plants that abound in your environment. Incorporate the herbs in your kitchen with your meals on a regular basis. Basil, rosemary, dill, turmeric, anise — all your favorite spices are herbs. Grow basil, cilantro and onions on your kitchen window sill. Herbs are foods that heal you.

If you have more space, build a planter bed. Begin to grow your own organic vegetables. Plant fruit trees — oranges, peaches, plums, lemons, cherries, apricots, apples, figs and persimmons — in your backyard. Raise your own goats or cows for fresh raw milk, cheeses, kefir and whey. Raise egg laying chickens for daily fresh organic eggs. Select different breeds of chickens that lay different colored eggs. Allow them to roam free to dig for insects. But protect your blueberries and low hanging fruits! I learned the hard way coming home to an empty bush after it was enjoyed by my chickens and foraging animal neighbors.

You are a positive force in your community. Grow your passion to help, lead and inspire others. Your desire to live to the fullest is exemplary and honorable. Your radiance will only continue to influence others positively as you improve your life and embody health. Continue to focus on the meals you have each day with family and friends gathered around the dinner table, for you are a beacon of light that will bring clarity into the world. As the health leader of those who follow you, I encourage you to take the next step forward. Health is an unfolding journey, not a final destination. I look forward to sharing the path with you. How about you bring the spring water and I provide the edible plant field guide? Together we will forage for the wild goodness nature provides us.

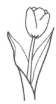

"Be the change you want to see in the world."

— Ghandi

To find a holistic health care practitioner, visit
www.thehealingbody.com

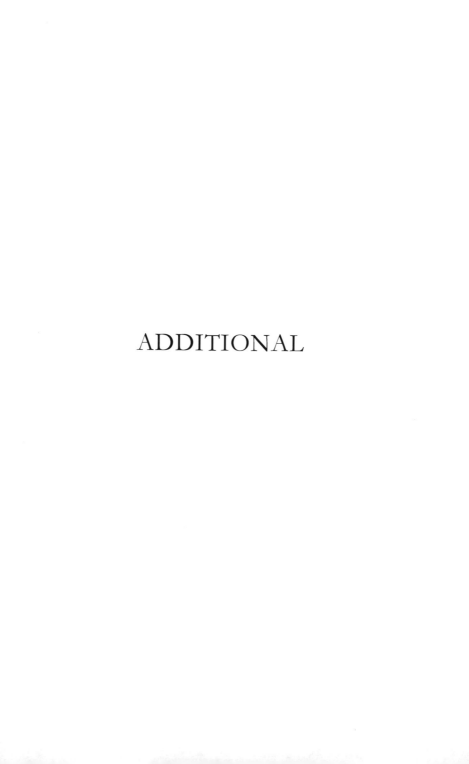

ADDITIONAL

OUR CHILDREN

"I know children regress after vaccination because it happened to my own son. Why aren't there any tests out there on the safety of how vaccines are administered in the real world, six at a time? Why have only two of the 36 shots our kids receive been looked at for their relationship to autism?"

— Jenny McCarthy

We have a responsibility to ensure we have healthy and happy children. They represent the radiant light and joy for all. Children will become our future leaders, innovators and inspiration. We must do what we can to maximize their health and thus their potential. While this book cannot address every cause of childhood diseases such as autism, learning disabilities and mood disorders (e.g., ADD and ADHD), they all have a connection to inadequate nutrition or systemic toxicity from our environment, including those caused by government mandated injections of foreign materials into fragile and developing bodies.

THE VACCINE ILLUSION

The theory behind vaccinations is to expose a child to a pathogen that induces their immune system to generate antibodies prior to a "real" exposure. Once the immune system has developed antibodies, there is a memory imprint that allows it to mount a rapid and sufficient immune response if the child were ever exposed to that pathogen again.

All doctors who have studied the basics of the immune system know that infants have absolutely no capacity to produce antibodies in their first year of life. Some hold that a child's own immune system is not fully functional until the age of three. Despite the understanding of an infant's basic physiological functions and limitations, the medical establishment recommends a total of 19 shots, containing 24 vaccines, to infants at 2, 4 and 6 months of age.[215]

A teacher and mentor of mine, Dr. Michael Gaeta lectured nationally for several years to holistic health care practitioners about the risks and dangers of vaccines. He was invited to speak at a national conference and created quite a stir by presenting the evidence that vaccines are completely pointless within the first 12 months after birth.

Later on that same day, Dr. Gaeta sat on a panel of experts to answer questions from conference attendees. Many of the questions were directed at a PhD immunologist on the panel, asking if the statements Dr. Gaeta had made in the morning presentation were true. To everyone's surprise, the immunologist confirmed every assertion he had made.

One attendee in the audience asked the following question to the highly respected immunologist on the panel. Her response is disturbing:[216]

Attendee: So, the science seems fairly clear that for the first year of life, probably, that the immunization is not stimulating the kind of response we expect it to stimulate.

Immunologist: True.

Attendee: So what's the rationale for continuing to do that if it's not doing what it's supposed to be [doing]?

Immunologist The vaccines are given at pediatric wellness visits, and the idea is that you are training the parent to bring their child in at all the pediatric wellness visits, and that it's only the year visit that actually is truly important. But for most parents you are not going to get them to bring their kid in if they don't come in at two months, four months and six months. And so it's actually more of a training thing. [crowd gasps]

Immunologist (con't): It was interesting when I was on the phone with the county public health department last week, with one of their vaccine nurses. She was like, 'Oh, you're talking about vaccines? Make sure you tell them they have to do that year shot because the first three [the 2, 4 and 6 month shots] don't work.' I was like, 'Yeah, I know.' [laughter].

The actual audio recording of this dialogue can be found on www.gaetacommunications.com.

The term "immunization" is a misnomer. Its definition is "resistance to infection to a particular pathogen." The FDA mandates that all pharmaceutical drugs be tested against a placebo to verify efficacy. That means in clinical trials with a significant number of test subjects, the drug must create a substantial positive effect on an ill population. This benefit must be significantly greater than the positive effect of a sugar pill to prove that the drug is efficacious.

Vaccines have never been subject to this requirement. Unfortunately, no vaccine has ever been tested for efficacy against a placebo. In the field where "evidence based" research is the pride and joy of Western medicine, vaccinations are *assumed* to work.

I have heard countless horror stories from parents who vaccinated their children only to find that the child reacted unfavorably. The day after a mother brought her twin sons to their pediatrician for vaccinations, one of them stopped talking. She returned to the doctor and demanded answers. His response: "It's just a coincidence. We'll run more tests on him to investigate what is going on." This poor boy has not spoken for three years and the mother knew better than to subject her son to invasive machinery because she *knew* what the cause was. The prescribing medical doctor failed to admit that it could be the vaccine.

The evening after, another couple brought their daughter for vaccinations and she experienced a succession of seizures. The next day, the doctor nonchalantly reported, "It's just a coincidence. Let's wait a few days to see if it happens again." The parents were infuriated.

It is not uncommon for seizures to occur after a Hepatitis B or DTP (Diphtheria, Tetanus, Acellular Pertussis) vaccine.[217,218,219,220] So when parents begin to ask what in a vaccine would cause a child to become mute or have uncontrollable seizures, we find ingredients that are quite toxic.

- **Aluminum:** a known neurotoxin that has been associated with Alzheimer's disease, dementia and seizures.
- **Thimerosal:** a salt derived from mercury used as a disinfectant and preservative; has been linked to brain and kidney damage, as well as immune and neurological disorders.[221,222,223]
- **Formaldehyde:** a known cancer-causing chemical;[224] used to "inactivate" viruses and detoxify bacterial toxins; has also been shown to be injurious to multiple organs (pancreas, liver, fallopian tubes) and to trigger gene mutations.[225,226]
- **Carbolic Acid (Phenol):** believed to cause gender mutation; a deadly poison used as a disinfectant and dye.
- **Antibiotics:** neomycin, streptomycin and a variety of other drugs to which increasing numbers of the population are demonstrating serious allergies, and to which increasing numbers of microbes are developing genetically transmitted tolerance.
- **Acetone:** used in fingernail polish remover and as a solvent.
- **Alum:** used as a preservative.
- **Other toxic chemicals**: traces of other chemicals such as sodium hydroxide, sorbitol, hydrolyzed gelatin, benzethonium chloride, methylparaben — some of which are known to or suspected of causing cancer.

The harmful contents of vaccines are overwhelming for the body to deal with. Little is known about the long-term side effects from injecting these harmful substances. In Part I of this book, we saw that side effects to pharmaceuticals do not always occur right away. Many can take years to develop. The same applies for vaccines.

Informative vaccine related documentaries are available. *Shots in the Dark* is produced by mothers of children who experienced debilitating side effects immediately after the injection of various vaccines. An excellent book that thoroughly documents the history and development of vaccinations as a method of generating additional revenue for the pharmaceutical giants is *The Vaccine Illusion* by Tetyana Obukhanych.

MOTHER'S MILK IS MAGICAL

A mother's breast milk is the perfect food for a newborn and growing infant. The only time it becomes unacceptable is when the mother undergoes chemotherapy or is exposed to other highly toxic chemicals. Unfortunately, most commercial infant formula manufacturers market their products so consumers incorrectly believe they are nearly as nutritive as breast milk. Nestlé's advertisements for their commercial Good Start® formula states, "We learned from the best, so we could give your baby our best. Nothing else is breast milk. Nothing else is Good Start." Pharmaceutical companies are the manufacturers of many other infant formulas. Abbott Laboratories markets the Similac® infant formula brand. Bristol Myers Squibb used to own a portion of Mead Johnson Nutrition Co. which markets Enfamil®. Bristol Myers Squibb split off its holdings in Mead Johnson Nutrition Co. to deliver value to its shareholders.[227]

Infants who are not breastfed show an increased incidence of infectious morbidity, including otitis media (ear infections), gastroenteritis and pneumonia, as well as elevated risks of childhood obesity, type 1 and type 2 diabetes, leukemia and sudden infant death syndrome (SIDS).[228,229, 230, 231, 232, 233, 234, 235, 236] Feeding infant formula to newborns is associated with lower I.Q.s and increased allergies.[237,238,239] Infant formulas also increase a baby girl's risk of developing breast cancer later in life.[240]

Just as whole food nutrition is important for adults, the whole milk from a mother is key to the health of her child. Poor lactation indicates that a mother's health is compromised. A mother who experiences challenges producing sufficient amounts of breast milk should seek the help of a holistic health care practitioner and lactation consultant. They will be able to identify the cause of insufficient lactation to ensure her child has sufficient nutrition for a growing body.

In situations where a child is adopted, a local breast milk bank is not yet established or for whatever reason, accessibility to a holistic health care practitioner is impossible, excellent homemade infant formula recipes and guidelines on properly nourishing a growing baby are provided in *Super Nutrition for Babies* by Katherine Erlich, MD and Kelly Genzlinger, CNC.

THE SEDATION OF THE NEXT GENERATION

As I was writing this book, I took a flight from Florida to California. Next to me sat a mother and her baby daughter of 14 months who began to cry as soon as I sat down. I apologized because I had thought I made a mistake and took her seat. However, it turned out that she had missed her naptime. Furthermore, cramped airplane seats and change in cabin pressure made it difficult for her to fall asleep. The mother apologized for her child's bellows of agony, but I assured her that it was not an issue for me because I am a future father. A child expressing discomfort is entirely normal. I simply returned to my laptop and continued typing away on the next chapter.

After a few minutes, the mother reached into her carry-on luggage and pulled out a bottle of liquid Benadryl®, an over the counter drug used to suppress allergy symptoms with sedation as a known side effect. I watched her administer a syringe full of Benadryl® to the child. Afterward, she turned to me and said, "Oh, it's okay. The pediatrician diagnosed her with allergies." I never did question her intention to feed her baby a syringe full of Benadryl®, nor did I have a response to her statement. I remained quiet and in awe that our society has taught its parents to administer pharmaceutical drugs to sedate children.

In that moment I realized that parents use pharmacology to mandate certain behaviors just as psychiatrists prescribe antidepressants to suppress a child's natural vocalization of hunger or tiredness.

The issue extends beyond a screaming child or a mother who feels shame among a crowd of strangers. While some may become annoyed that a crying baby is on board disrupting their travel slumber or quiet reading, we were all once a young baby. At some point in our infant lives, as a baby who missed a nap, we cried as if the world was about to end. Did our mother drug us to sleep?

Let us practice compassion for mothers and their crying children — sparing their developing liver and kidneys from biochemical trauma. We must endeavor to protect the future generations and safeguard their opportunity to live a healthy life by fully expressing their genetic potential. They are the shining light that leads us to a brighter future. If we can provide them a safe haven at the local playground as well as the global airways, we can surely provide them a heaven on earth.

21 QUESTIONS TO ASK

<u>Questions to ask your allopathic medical doctor:</u>
1) Are the specific pharmaceutical medications you are prescribing addictive?
2) Do you have any experience helping patients come off addictive pharmaceuticals?
3) What are the known side effects for each of the prescribed medications?
4) Do any of the prescribed medications inhibit my liver and kidney's ability to excrete toxins or increase the level of physical stress on my detoxification organs?
5) Is this pharmaceutical drug you are prescribing known to cause another disease?
6) Is the pharmaceutical drug you are prescribing me known to cause death?
7) For any health issue or out of range lab value, ask: Which organs need help and what can you do to regenerate them?
8) Have you ever been bought out? Let me rephrase that, have you ever gone out for dinner with a pharmaceutical sales representative and allowed them to foot the bill?
9) If a medical doctor prescribes a poison for a child (or adult), who can diagnose him or her with Münchausen Syndrome by Proxy?

Questions to ask your holistic health care practitioner:

1) Have you studied the work and findings of Dr. Weston Price which attribute the cause of all cavities, disease and degeneration to malnutrition?

2) Are you familiar with Dr. Page's Food Plan and how to restore proper mineral ratios for a healthy body?

3) Where is your favorite farmer's market?

4) Do you stay abreast with the information provided on Dr. Joseph Mercola's website?

5) Are you aware that the use of synthetic vitamins in high dosages is pharmacology?

6) Are you trained in how to use the whole food concentrates created by Dr. Royal Lee?

7) Are you capable of identifying which organs are negatively impacted by pesticides or other chemicals and how to use whole food concentrates to support the body's ability to properly detoxify them out?

Questions to ask yourself:

1) Who is my holistic health care practitioner?

2) Do I have a catastrophic health insurance policy to provide coverage for emergency and hospital related services?

3) Am I ready to upgrade my diet to ensure my body has the raw building blocks to repair itself?

4) Am I ready to enhance the removal of toxins from my body with the support of a purification program?

5) Am I ready to support my healing body?

ACKNOWLEDGMENTS

This book, like most projects, was a collective effort. My wife provided logistical, emotional and intellectual support. I thank my brother, for being there for me and for being the heroic firefighter that he is. I thank my sister and father, for always reminding me that patience with life changes is a must. These people continually inspire me with their commitment to life and to love. I am profoundly privileged to share my life with them.

For the amazing imagery that captured the concept of the content and the eyes of the readers, I thank Raymond Lee, John Ferguson II, and Ulysses Galgo for their creative spirit in manifesting an enchanting book cover. I thank David Rotman for his simple and sophisticated icons that fit perfectly into every chapter.

Heavy editorial lifting was shared by my talented friends Ken Liu, Paul Wang and Jovi Cotio. Support to polish a diamond in the rough came from their keen perception and deep understanding on the subject matter, which have contributed marvelously to the book's fruition. I thank my friends and colleagues who read the manuscript at various stages and made so many fine suggestions. In particular I thank Amanda Diuzniewski, Sara Ortega, Carl Dimailig, Justin Toal, Yvonne Franklin, Paul Cornelius, David Carroll Carr and Sherry Granader who gave detailed attention to the manuscript and whose reflections have been invaluable. This book would not be what it is without their honesty and clarity.

While an author traditionally does not thank people quoted in his book, accuracy and respect require special thanks to three groups: the pioneers, especially Royal Lee, Melvin Page, Francis Pottenger, Weston A. Price and Harvey Wiley, who did everything and gave their all to provide humanity the opportunity to heal with food; the contemporary teachers who pass on the teachings of the pioneers, especially Michael Gaeta, Michael Dobbins, Holly Carling, Michael Greer, Kerry Bone, Lee Carroll, Ronda Nelson, Jay Robbins, Don Lawson, Marlene Merritt, Freddie Ulan, Stuart White, Mark Anderson at Selene River Press, and John Brady at the International Foundation for Nutrition and Health who encourage their students to inspire patients; the amazing holistic healers I work with. Because of your willingness to wholeheartedly spread health and wellness, I am inspired to share my story and experience. May you continue to educate and implement whole food nutrition to motivate your patients, friends and family to bring the focus back to the table where joyful laughter and colorful food serve as the real nourishment for the healing body, mind and soul.

Lastly, I thank you, dear reader, for joining me in the search for a way of life that finds health in honoring the human spirit and our interdependence with one another and the whole earth community.

BOOKS AND RESOURCES

Drug-Induced Diseases by L. Meyler and H.M. Peck

Drug-Induced Diseases: Prevention, Detection, and Management, 2nd Edition by Dr. James E. Tisdale, Pharm.D. and Douglas A. Miller, Pharm.D.

Iodine: Why You Need It, Why You Can't Live Without It (4th Edition by David Brownstein, MD

Overdosed America, The Broken Promise of American Medicine by John Abramson, MD

The Cholesterol Myth: Exposing the Fallacy That Saturated Fat and Cholesterol Cause Heart Disease by Uffe Ravnskov, MD

Your Body's Many Cries for Water by F. Batmanghelidj, MD

Deep Nutrition: Why Your Genes Need Traditional Food by Catherine Shanahan, MD

Nutrition and Physical Degeneration by Weston A. Price, DDS

Folk Medicine by D.C. Jarvis, MD

Seeds of Deception, by Jeffrey M. Smith

The Real Truth about Vitamins and Anti-oxidants by Judith Decava, CNC

Applied Protomorphology by Royal Lee, DDS

Good Calories, Bad Calories by Gary Taubes

Primal Diet by Aajonus Vonderplanitz

Nourishing Traditions by Sally Fallon

Rawvolution by Cherie Soria

Drug-Induced Nutrient Depletion Handbook by Ross Pelton, James B. LaValle and Ernest B. Hawkins

Know Your Fats by Mary Enig, PhD

Primal Body Primal Mind by Nora Gedgaudas, CNS, CNT

Wild Fermentation by Sandor Katz

The Vegetarian Myth by Lierre Keith

Clinical Purification: A Complete Treatment and Reference Manual by Gina Nick, ND

The Vaccine Illusion by Tetyana Obukhanych, PhD

Super Nutrition for Babies by Katherine Erlich, MD and Kelly Genzlinger, CNC.

ONLINE RESOURCES

www.thehealingbody.com
www.westonaprice.org
www.drroyallee.com
www.seleneriverpress.com
www.ifnh.org
www.mercola.com
www.responsibletechnology.org
www.standardprocess.com
www.price-pottenger.org
www.eatlocal.com
www.localharvest.org
www.findaspring.com
www.epocrates.com
www.pubmed.gov

NOTES

[1] Jukes TH. The prevention and conquest of scurvy, beri-beri, and pellagra. Prev, Med. 1989 Nov;18(6):877-83.

[2] Garland CF, Garland FC, Gorham ED, Lipkin M, Newmark H, Mohr SB, Holick MF. The role of vitamin D in cancer prevention. Am J Public Health. 2006, Feb;96(2):252-61.

[3] Schwartz GG. Vitamin D and intervention trials in prostate cancer: from theory to therapy. Ann Epidemiol. 2009 Feb;19(2):96-102.

[4] Holick MF. Vitamin D: its role in cancer prevention and treatment. Prog Biophys Mol Biol. 2006 Sep;92(1):49-59. Epub 2006 Mar 10.

[5] National Health and Nutrition Examination Survey (NHANES) 2003–2006 and 2007–2008.

[6] Murray C, Kulkarni S, Ezzati M. Eight Americas: new perspectives on U.S. health disparities. *American Journal of Preventive Medicine, 2005*, 29:4–10.

[7] CDC 2011 National Diabetes Fact Sheet http://www.cdc.gov/diabetes/pubs/pdf/ndfs_2011.pdf, Accessed July 9, 2012.

[8] Eyre H, Kahn R, Robertson RM, Clark NG, Doyle C, Hong Y, Gansler T, Glynn T, Smith RA, Taubert K, Thun MJ; American Cancer Society; American Diabetes Association; American Heart Association. Preventing cancer, cardiovascular disease, and diabetes: a common agenda for the American Cancer Society, the American Diabetes Association, and the American Heart Association. Stroke. 2004 Aug; 35(8): 1999-2010.

[9] Cancer Facts & Figures, http://www.cancer.org/acs/groups/content/@epidemiologysurveilance/documents/document/acspc-031941.pdf, Accessed July 9, 2012.

[10] Circulation.2012; 125: 188-197 http://circ.ahajournals.org/content/125/1/188.full.pdf+html, Accessed July 9, 2012.

[11] FDA.gov AERS.

[12] The U.S. Health System in Perspective: A Comparison of Twelve Industrialized Nations http://www.commonwealthfund.org/~/media/Files/Publications/Issue%20Brief/2011/Jul/1532_Squires_US_hlt_sys_comparison_12_nations_intl_brief_v2.pdf, Accessed July 6, 2012.

[13] Commonwealth Fund 2010 International Health Policy Survey of Eleven Countries.

[14] Systematic overview of warfarin and its drug and food interactions". *Arch. Intern. Med.* 165 (10): 1095–106.

[15] Ivarsson U, Nilsson H, Santesson J, Eds. *A FOA briefing book on chemical weapons: threat, effects, and protection.* Umeå, National Defense Research Establishment, 1992.

[16] Einhorn J. Nitrogen mustard: the origin of chemotherapy for cancer. Int J Radiat Oncol Biol Phys. 1985 Jul; 11(7): 1375-8.

[17] IARC Monographs on the Evaluation of Carcinogenic Risks to Humans, Overall Evaluations of Carcinogenicity: An Updating of IARC Monographs Volumes 1 to 42, http://monographs.iarc.fr/ENG/Monographs/suppl7/suppl7.pdf, Accessed July 11, 2012.

[18] Gagnadoux F, Hureaux J, Vecellio L, Urban T, Le Pape A, Valo I, Montharu J, Leblond V, Boisdron-Celle M, Lerondel S, Majoral C, Diot P, Racineux JL, Lemarie E. Aerosolized chemotherapy. J Aerosol Med Pulm Drug Deliv. 2008 Mar;21(1):61-70.

[19] Paskulin GA, Gazzola Zen PR, de Camargo Pinto LL, Rosa R, Graziadio C. Combined chemotherapy and teratogenicity. Birth Defects Res A Clin Mol Teratol. 2005 Sep;73(9):634-7.

[20] Selig BP, Furr JR, Huey RW, Moran C, Alluri VN, Medders GR, Mumm CD, Hallford HG, Mulvihill JJ. Cancer chemotherapeutic agents as human teratogens. Birth Defects Res A Clin Mol Teratol. 2012 Aug;94(8):626-50.

[21] Abel U. Chemotherapy of advanced epithelial cancer--a critical review. Biomed Pharmacother. 1992; 46(10): 439-52.

[22] Peto J, Easton D. Cancer treatment trials--past failures, current progress and future prospects. Cancer Surv. 1989;8(3): 511-33.

[23] Anand P, Kunnumakkara AB, Sundaram C, Harikumar KB, Tharakan ST, Lai OS, Sung B, Aggarwal BB. Cancer is a preventable disease that requires major lifestyle changes. Pharm Res. 2008 Sep;25(9):2097-116. doi: 10.1007/s11095-008-9661-9. Epub 2008 Jul 15. Review. Erratum in: Pharm Res. 2008 Sep;25(9):2200. Kunnumakara, Ajaikumar B [corrected to Kunnumakkara, Ajaikumar B].

[24] Weisburger JH. Lifestyle, health and disease prevention: the underlying mechanisms. Eur J Cancer Prev. 2002 Aug;11 Suppl 2:S1-7.

[25] Tonks A. Withdrawal from paroxetine can be severe, warns FDA. BMJ. 2002 Feb 2;324(7332):260.

[26] Benazzi F. Venlafaxine withdrawal symptoms. Can J Psychiatry. 1996 Sep;41(7):487.

[27] Abdy NA, Gerhart K. Duloxetine Withdrawal Syndrome in a Newborn. Clin Pediatr (Phila). 2012 Jun 19.

[28] Scott HD, Rosebaum SE, Waters WJ, et al. Rhode Island Physicians' recognition and reporting of adverse drug reactions RIMed J. 1987; 70:311-316.

[29] David W. Bates, Drugs and Adverse Drug Reactions: How Worried Should We Be? JAMA.1998; 279(15): 1216-1217.

[30] Wysowski DK, Swartz L. Adverse drug event surveillance and drug withdrawals in the United States, 1969-2002: the importance of reporting suspected reactions. Arch Intern Med. 2005 Jun 27; 165(12): 1363-9.

[31] Food and drug administration (FDA) *FDA science and mission at risk: report of the Subcommittee on Science and Technology.* Available at: http://www.fda.gov/ohrms/dockets/ac/07/briefing/2007-4329b_02_01_FDA%20Report%20on%20Science%20and%20Technology.pdf, Accessed July 4, 2012.

[32] Donaldson L, Philip P. Patient safety: a global priority. *Bulletin of the World Health Organization* 2004, 82:892−893.

[33] Meier RP, Perneger TV, Stern R, Rizzoli R, Peter RE. Increasing Occurrence of Atypical Femoral Fractures Associated With Bisphosphonate Use Atypical Femoral Fractures and Bisphosphonate Use. Arch Intern Med. 2012 Jun 25; 172(12): 930-6.

[34] Akintoye SO, Hersh EV. Risks for jaw osteonecrosis drastically increases after 2 years of bisphosphonate therapy. J Evid Based Dent Pract. 2012 Jun; 12(2): 116-8.

[35] Peat ID, Healy S, Reid DM, and Ralston SH. Steroid induced osteoporosis: an opportunity for prevention? Ann Rheum Dis. 1995 Jan; 54(1): 66-8.

[36] Hugues FC, Gourlot C, Le Jeunne C. [Drug-induced gynecomastia]. Ann Med Interne (Paris). 2000 Feb;151(1):10-7.

[37] Tanner LA, Bosco LA. Gynecomastia associated with calcium channel blocker therapy. Arch Intern Med. 1988 Feb;148(2):379-80.

[38] Lee WM. Acute liver failure. Semin Respir Crit Care Med. 2012 Feb; 33(1): 36-45. Epub 2012 Mar 23.

[39] Chun LJ, Tong MJ, Busuttil RW, Hiatt JR. Acetaminophen hepatotoxicity and acute liver failure. J Clin Gastroenterol. 2009 Apr; 43(4): 342-9.

[40] Lai DP, Ren XH, Yao JP, Liu ML, Xu G, Chen ZJ, Ling GL. [Study on the effect using hemoperfusion to treat tylenol poisoned patients]. Zhonghua Lao Dong WeiSheng Zhi Ye Bing Za Zhi. 2012 Apr;30(4):310-2.

[41] Bailey B, Amre DK, Gaudreault P. Fulminant hepatic failure secondary to acetaminophen poisoning: a systematic review and meta-analysis of prognostic criteria determining the need for liver transplantation. Crit Care Med. 2003 Jan;31(1):299-305.

[42] Ranganathan SS, Sathiadas MG, Sumanasena S, Fernandopulle M, Lamabadusuriya SP, Fernandopulle BM. Fulminant hepatic failure and paracetamol overuse with therapeutic intent in febrile children. Indian J Pediatr. 2006 Oct;73(10):871-5.

[43] Walsh TS, Wigmore SJ, Hopton P, Richardson R, Lee A. Energy expenditure in acetaminophen-induced fulminant hepatic failure. Crit Care Med. 2000 Mar;28(3):649-54.

[44] Furukawa F, Yoshimasu T. Animal models of spontaneous and drug-induced cutaneous lupus erythematosus. *Autoimmunity Reviews.* 2005;4(6):345–350.

[45] Yoon J, Lee SH, Kim TH, Choi DJ, Kim JP, Yoon TJ. Concurrence of Stevens-Johnson Syndrome and Bilateral Parotitis after Minocycline Therapy. Case Rep Dermatol. 2010 Jun 1;2(2):88-94.

[46] A. V. Marzano, P. Vezzoli, and C. Crosti, "Drug-induced lupus: an update on its dermatologic aspects," Lupus, vol. 18, no. 11, pp. 935–940, 2009.

[47] C. D. Vedove, M. Del Giglio, D. Schena, and G. Girolomoni, "Drug-induced lupus erythematosus," Archives of Dermatological Research, vol. 301, no. 1, pp. 99–105, 2009.

[48] A. Mounach, M. Ghazi, A. Nouijai et al., "Drug-induced lupus-like syndrome in ankylosing spondylitis treated with infliximab," Clinical and Experimental Rheumatology, vol. 26, no. 6, pp. 1116–1118, 2008.

[49] M. Debandt, O. Vittecoq, V. Descamps, X. Le Loët, and O. Meyer, "Anti-TNF-α-induced systemic lupus syndrome," Clinical Rheumatology, vol. 22, no. 1, pp. 56–61, 2003.

[50] Krouse RS, Royal RE, Heywood G, Weintraub BD, White DE, Steinberg SM, Rosenberg SA, Schwartzentruber DJ. Thyroid dysfunction in 281 patients with metastatic melanoma or renal carcinoma treated with interleukin-2 alone. J Immunother Emphasis Tumor Immunol. 1995 Nov;18(4):272-8.

[51] Batcher EL, Tang XC, Singh BN, Singh SN, Reda DJ, Hershman JM; SAFE-T Investigators. Thyroid function abnormalities during amiodarone therapy for persistent atrial fibrillation. Am J Med. 2007 Oct;120(10):880-5.

[52] Drucker D, Eggo MC, Salit IE, Burrow GN. Ethionamide-induced goitrous hypothyroidism. Ann Intern Med. 1984 Jun;100(6):837-9.

[53] McDonnell ME, Braverman LE, Bernardo J. Hypothyroidism due to ethionamide. N Engl J Med. 2005 Jun 30;352(26):2757-9.

[54] Dalgard O, Bjøro K, Hellum K, Myrvang B, Bjøro T, Haug E, Bell H. Thyroid dysfunction during treatment of chronic hepatitis C with interferon alpha: no association with either interferon dosage or efficacy of therapy. J Intern Med. 2002 May;251(5):400-6.

[55] Eyal O, Rose SR. Autoimmune thyroiditis during leuprolide acetate treatment. J Pediatr. 2004 Mar;144(3):394-6.

[56] Bocchetta A, Mossa P, Velluzzi F, Mariotti S, Zompo MD, Loviselli A. Ten-year follow-up of thyroid function in lithium patients. J Clin Psychopharmacol. 2001 Dec;21(6):594-8.

[57] Maayan-Metzger A, Sack J, Mazkereth R, Vardi A, Kuint J. Somatostatin treatment of congenital chylothorax may induce transient hypothyroidism in newborns. Acta Paediatr. 2005 Jun;94(6):785-9.

[58] Liappas J, Paparrigopoulos T, Mourikis I, Soldatos C. Hypothyroidism induced by quetiapine: a case report. J Clin Psychopharmacol. 2006 Apr;26(2):208-9.

[59] Kim DL, Song KH, Lee JH, Lee KY, Kim SK. Rifampin-induced hypothyroidism without underlying thyroid disease. Thyroid. 2007 Aug;17(8):793-5.

[60] Travis LB, Andersson M, Gospodarowicz M, van Leeuwen FE, Bergfeldt K, Lynch CF, Curtis RE, Kohler BA, Wiklund T, Storm H, Holowaty E, Hall P, Pukkala E, Sleijfer DT, Clarke EA, Boice JD Jr, Stovall M, Gilbert E., J Natl Cancer Inst. 2000 Jul 19;92(14):1165-71.

[61] Leone G, Pagano L, Ben-Yehuda D, Voso MT. Therapy-related leukemia and myelodysplasia: susceptibility and incidence. Haematologica. 2007 Oct;92(10):1389-98.

[62] Tebbi CK, London WB, Friedman D, Villaluna D, De Alarcon PA, Constine LS, Mendenhall NP, Sposto R, Chauvenet A, Schwartz CL. Dexrazoxane-associated risk for acute myeloid leukemia/myelodysplastic syndrome and other secondary malignancies in pediatric Hodgkin's disease. J Clin Oncol. 2007 Feb 10;25(5):493-500.

[63] Campone M, Roché H, Kerbrat P, Bonneterre J, Romestaing P, Fargeot P, Namer M,Monnier A, Montcuquet P, Goudier MJ, Fumoleau P. Secondary leukemia after epirubicin-based adjuvant chemotherapy in operable breast cancer patients: 16 years experience of the French Adjuvant Study Group. Ann Oncol. 2005 Aug;16(8):1343-51. Epub 2005 May 19.

[64] Smith MA, Rubinstein L, Anderson JR, Arthur D, Catalano PJ, Freidlin B, Heyn R, Khayat A, Krailo M, Land VJ, Miser J, Shuster J, Vena D. Secondary leukemia or myelodysplastic syndrome after treatment with epipodophyllotoxins. J Clin Oncol. 1999 Feb;17(2):569-77.

[65] Kröger N, Damon L, Zander AR, Wandt H, Derigs G, Ferrante P, Demirer T, Rosti G; Solid Tumor Working Party of the European Group for Blood and Marrow Transplantation; German Adjuvant Breast Cancer Study Group; University of California, San Francisco. Secondary acute leukemia following mitoxantrone-based high-dose chemotherapy for primary breast cancer patients. Bone Marrow Transplant. 2003 Dec;32(12):1153-7.

[66] Cantarovich M, Durrbach A, Hiesse C, Ladouceur M, Benoit G, Charpentier B. 20-year follow-up results of a randomized controlled trial comparing antilymphocyte globulin induction to no induction in renal transplant patients. Transplantation. 2008 Dec 27; 86(12):1732-7.

[67]Hiesse C, Kriaa F, Rieu P, Larue JR, Benoit G, Bellamy J, Blanchet P, Charpentier B. Incidence and type of malignancies occurring after renal transplantation in conventionally and cyclosporine-treated recipients: analysis of a 20-year period in 1600 patients. Transplant Proc. 1995 Feb;27(1):972-4.

[68] Dantal J, Hourmant M, Cantarovich D, Giral M, Blancho G, Dreno B, Soulillou JP. Effect of long-term immunosuppression in kidney-graft recipients on cancer

incidence: randomised comparison of two cyclosporin regimens. Lancet. 1998 Feb 28;351(9103):623-8.

[69] Swinnen LJ, Costanzo-Nordin MR, Fisher SG, O'Sullivan EJ, Johnson MR, Heroux AL, Dizikes GJ, Pifarre R, Fisher RI. Increased incidence of lymphoproliferative disorder after immunosuppression with the monoclonal antibody OKT3 in cardiac-transplant recipients. N Engl J Med. 1990 Dec 20;323(25):1723-8.

[70] Opelz G, Döhler B. Lymphomas after solid organ transplantation: a collaborative transplant study report. Am J Transplant. 2004 Feb;4(2):222-30.

[71] Frei U, Bode U, Repp H, Schindler R, Brunkhorst R, Vogt P, Hauss J, Pichlmayr R. Malignancies under cyclosporine after kidney transplantation: analysis of a 10-year period. Transplant Proc. 1993 Feb;25(1 Pt 2):1394-6.

[72] Banks E, Beral V, Bull D, et al. Breast cancer and hormone-replacement therapy in the Million Women Study. Lancet. 2003;362:419-427.

[73] Chlebowski RT, Hendrix SL, Langer RD, Stefanick ML, Gass M, Lane D, Rodabough RJ, Gilligan MA, Cyr MG, Thomson CA, Khandekar J, Petrovitch H, McTiernan A; WHI Investigators. Influence of estrogen plus progestin on breast cancer and mammography in healthy postmenopausal women: the Women's Health Initiative Randomized Trial. JAMA. 2003 Jun 25;289(24):3243-53.

[74] Hammond CB, Jelovsek FR, Lee KL, Creasman WT, Parker RT. Effects of long-term estrogen replacement therapy. II. Neoplasia. Am J Obstet Gynecol. 1979 Mar 1;133(5):537–547.

[75] Fisher B, Costantino JP, Wickerham DL, Redmond CK, Kavanah M, Cronin WM, Vogel V, Robidoux A, Dimitrov N, Atkins J, Daly M, Wieand S, Tan-Chiu E, Ford L, Wolmark N. Tamoxifen for prevention of breast cancer: report of the National Surgical Adjuvant Breast and Bowel Project P-1 Study. J Natl Cancer Inst. 1998 Sep 16;90(18):1371-88.

[76] Knight A, Askling J, Granath F, et al. Urinary bladder cancer in Wegener's granulomatosis: risks and relation to cyclophosphamide. Ann Rheum Dis. 2004;63:1307-1311.

[77] Schairer C, Lubin J, Troisi R, Sturgeon S, Brinton L, Hoover R. Menopausal estrogen and estrogen-progestin replacement therapy and breast cancer risk. JAMA. 2000 Jan 26; 283(4): 485-91. Erratum in: JAMA 2000 Nov 22-29; 284(20): 2597.

[78] Brinton LA, Lamb EJ, Moghissi KS, Scoccia B, Althuis MD, Mabie JE, Westhoff CL. Ovarian cancer risk after the use of ovulation-stimulating drugs. Obstet Gynecol. 2004 Jun;103(6):1194-203.

[79] Clinical therapeutics and the Recognition of Drug-Induced Disease, A MedWatch Continuing Education Article, June 1995, http://www.fda.gov/downloads/Safety/MedWatch/UCM168515.pdf, Last accessed May 2, 2013.

[80] Orkin FK. Error in medicine. JAMA. 1995 Aug 9; 274(6): 459-60; author reply 460-1.

[81] Vincent C, Stanhope N, and Crowley-Murphy M. Reasons for not reporting adverse incidents: an empirical study. J Eval Clin Pract. 1999 Feb; 5(1): 13-21.

[82] Shojania KG, Duncan BW, McDonald KM, Wachter RM, Markowitz AJ. Making health care safer: a critical analysis of patient safety practices. Evid Rep Technol Assess (Summ). 2001;(43): I-x, 1-668.

[83] Kohn LT, Corrigan JM, Donaldson MS, Eds. *To err is human: building a safer health system. Washington, DC, National Academy Press, Committee on Quality of Health* Care in America, Institute of Medicine, 1999.

[84] Gary Null, PhD; Carolyn Dean MD, ND; Martin Feldman, MD; Debora Rasio, MD; and Dorothy Smith, PhD, Death by Medicine, Life Extension Magazine. March 2004 (http://www.lef.org/magazine/mag2004/mar2004_awsi_death_01.htm).

[85] ICD-10 Codes for Cause-Specific Healthy People 2010 Mortality Objectives (http://www.cdc.gov/nchs/data/hpdata2010/tracking_healthy_people/appendix _c.pdf) Accessed July, 13, 2012.

[86] Graham DJ, Ouellet-Hellstrom R, MaCurdy TE, Ali F, Sholley C, Worrall C, Kelman JA. Risk of acute myocardial infarction, stroke, heart failure, and death in elderly Medicare patients treated with rosiglitazone or pioglitazone. JAMA. 2010 Jul 28; 304(4): 411-8. Epub 2010 Jun 28.

[87] Alberts, et al., *Molecular Biology of the Cell: Fourth Edition*, New York: Garland Science, 2002, p. 588.

[88] Ohvo-Rekilä H, Ramstedt B, Leppimäki P, Slotte JP. Cholesterol interactions with phospholipids in membranes. Prog Lipid Res. 2002 Jan;41(1):66-97.

[89] Tymoczko, John L.; Stryer Berg Tymoczko; Stryer, Lubert; Berg, Jeremy Mark (2002).*Biochemistry*. San Francisco: W.H. Freeman. pp. 726–727.

[90] Hanukoglu I. Steroidogenic enzymes: structure, function, and role inregulation of steroid hormone biosynthesis. J Steroid Biochem Mol Biol. 1992Dec;43(8):779-804.

[91] Cranton, E M, MD, and J P Frackelton, MD, *Journal of Holistic Medicine*, Spring/Summer 1984, 6-37.

[92] Masterjohn C. The Many Functions of Cholesterol. http://www.cholesterol-and-health.com/. Published 2005. Accessed February 14, 2013.

[93] Engelberg, Hyman, *Lancet*, Mar 21, 1992, 339:727-728; Wood, W G, et al, *Lipids*, Mar 1999, 34(3):225-234.

[94] Pawlina W, Ross MW (2006). *Histology: a text and atlas: with correlated cell and molecular biology*. Philadelphia: Lippincott Wiliams & Wilkins. pp. 230.

[95] "Multiple Risk Factor Intervention Trial; Risk Factor Changes and Mortality Results," *JAMA*, September 24, 1982, 248:12:1465.

[96] Smith LL. Another cholesterol hypothesis: cholesterol as antioxidant. Free Radic Biol Med. 1991;11(1):47-61.

[97] Hanukoglu I. Steroidogenic enzymes: structure, function, and role in regulation of steroid hormone biosynthesis. J Steroid Biochem Mol Biol. 1992 Dec;43(8):779-804.

98 The Top Prescription Drugs of 2009 in the US: CNS Therapeutics Rank among Highest Grossing, Craig W. Lindsley, *ACS Chemical Neuroscience* 2010 *1* (6), 407-408.

99 The Top Prescription Drugs of 2010 in the United States: Antipsychotics Show Strong Growth, Craig W. Lindsley, *ACS Chemical Neuroscience* 2011 *2* (6), 276-277.

100 Reduced synthesis of coenzyme Q10 may cause statin related myopathy - a systematic review, Nielsen ML, Pareek M, Henriksen JE. Ugeskr Laeger. 2011 Nov 14; 173(46): 2943-2948. Danish.

101 Statin-associated myopathy with normal creatine kinase levels, Phillips PS, Haas RH, Bannykh S, Hathaway S, Gray NL, Kimura BJ, Vladutiu GD, England JD; Scripps Mercy Clinical Research Center. Ann Intern Med. 2002 Oct 1; 137(7): 581-5.

102 Lipid-lowering drugs and mitochondrial function: effects of HMG-CoA reductase inhibitors on serum ubiquinone and blood lactate/pyruvate ratio, De Pinieux G, Chariot P, Ammi-Saïd M, Louarn F, Lejonc JL, Astier A, Jacotot B, Gherardi R., Br J Clin Pharmacol. 1996 Sep; 42(3): 333-7.

103 Golomb BA, Evans MA. Statin adverse effects: a review of the literature and evidence for a mitochondrial mechanism. Am J Cardiovasc Drugs. 2008;8(6): 373-418.

104 Goldstein MR, Mascitelli L. Do Statins Cause Diabetes? Curr Diab Rep. 2013 Mar 2.

105 Newman TB, Hulley SB. Carcinogenicity of lipid lowering drugs. JAMA. 1996 Jan 3; 275(1): 55-60.

106 Carcinogenicity of lipid-lowering drugs. JAMA. 1996 May 15; 275(19): 1481-2.

107 Handbook of Kidney Transplantation by Gabriel M Danovitch.

108 M Jennings, JR Shortland, JL Maddocks. Interstitial nephritis associated with frusemide. JR Soc Med. 1986 April; 79(4): 239-240.

109 Magil AB, Ballon HS, Cameron EC, Rae A. Acute interstitial nephritis associated with thiazide diuretics. Clinical and pathologic observations in three cases. Am J Med. 1980 Dec;69(6):939-43.

110 Linton AL, Clark WF, Driedger AA, Turnbull DI, Lindsay RM. Acute interstitial nephritis due to drugs: Review of the literature with a report of nine cases. Ann Intern Med. 1980 Nov;93(5):735-41.

111 Mullick FG. Papillary necrosis, marked, associated with aspirin abuse and interstitial nephritis, acute and chronic. Mil Med. 1984 Oct;149(10):569, 575.

112 Scott Hensky, "As Drug Ad Spending Rises: A Look at Four Campaigns," Wall Street Journal, February 9, 2004.

113 See Scott Hensely, "When Doctors Go to Class, Industry Often Foots the Bill," *Wall Street Journal,* December 4, 2002.

114 ACCMEâ 2010 Annual Report Data.

115 M. Healy, "In Short, Marketing Works," Los Angeles Times, August 6, 2007.

[116] DeVoe J, Fryer Jr GE, Hargraves JL, Phillips RL, Green LA. Does career dissatisfaction affect the ability of family physicians to deliver high-quality patient care? J Fam Pract. 2002 Mar; 51(3): 223-8.

[117] "To Demonstrate "Basic 7" Diet, *The Free Lance-Star.* The Associated Press (Fredericksburg, Virginia). 2 April 1943. Retrieved 2 June 2011.

[118] Prival MJ, Peiperl MD, Bell SJ. Determination of combined benzidine in FD & C yellow no. 5 (tartrazine), using a highly sensitive analytical method. Food Chem Toxicol. 1993 Oct; 31(10): 751-8.

[119] Benzidine (Group 1), Evidence for carcinogenicity to humans (*sufficient*), http://www.inchem.org/documents/iarc/suppl7/benzidine.html, Accessed July 24, 2012.

[120] Ganguly R, Pierce GN. Trans fat involvement in cardiovascular disease. Mol Nutr Food Res. 2012 Jul; 56(7): 1090-6.

[121] Morris MC, Evans DA, Bienias JL, Tangney CC, Bennett DA, Aggarwal N, Schneider J, Wilson RS. Dietary fats and the risk of incident Alzheimer disease. Arch Neurol. 2003 Feb; 60(2): 194-200.

[122] Chavarro JE, Stampfer MJ, Campos H, Kurth T, Willett WC, Ma J. A prospective study of trans-fatty acid levels in blood and risk of prostate cancer. Cancer Epidemiol Biomarkers Prev. 2008 Jan; 17(1): 95-101.

[123] Kavanagh K, Jones KL, Sawyer J, Kelley K, Carr JJ, Wagner JD, Rudel LL. Trans fat diet induces abdominal obesity and changes in insulin sensitivity in monkeys. Obesity (Silver Spring). 2007 Jul; 15(7): 1675-84.

[124] Chavarro JE, Rich-Edwards JW, Rosner BA, Willett WC. Dietary fatty acid intakes and the risk of ovulatory infertility. Am J Clin Nutr. 2007 Jan; 85(1): 231-7.

[125] Jensen J. Aspartame – The World's Best Ant Poison. *The Idaho Observer.* June 2006.

[126] Belpoggi F, Soffritti M, Padovani M, Degli Esposti D, Lauriola M, Minardi F. Results of long-term carcinogenicity bioassay on Sprague-Dawley rats exposed to aspartame administered in feed. Ann N Y Acad Sci. 2006 Sep;1076:559-77.

[127] Drug-Induced Nutrient Depletion Handbook, 2nd Edition, 2001, pg. 10.

[128] CS Johnston, CA Gaas. Vinegar: Medicinal Uses and Antiglycemic Effect, *MedGenMed,* 8(2): 61. May 30 2006.

[129] POTTENGER FM Jr. The effect of heat-processed foods and metabolized vitamin D milk on the dentofacial structures of experimental animals. Am J Orthod Oral Surg. 1946 Aug;32:467-85.

[130] Center for Disease Control and Prevention http://www.cdc.gov/nchs/fastats/fertile.htm, Accessed Aug 1, 2012.

[131] Center for Disease Control and Prevention, http://www.cdc.gov/reproductivehealth/Infertility/index.htm, Accessed Aug 1, 2012.

[132] Vikis HG, Gelman AE, Franklin A, Stein L, Rymaszewski A, Zhu J, Liu P, Tichelaar JW, Krupnick AS, You M. Neutrophils are required for 3 methylcholanthrene-initiated, butylated hydroxytoluene-promoted lung carcinogenesis. Mol Carcinog. 2011 Oct 17.

[133] Shearn CT, Fritz KS, Thompson JA. Protein damage from electrophiles and oxidants in lungs of mice chronically exposed to the tumor promoter butylated hydroxytoluene. Chem Biol Interact. 2011 Jul 15;192(3):278-86. Epub 2011 Apr 21.

[134] Wiley, Harvey W., M.D., *The History of a Crime Against the Food Law: The Amazing Story of the National Food and Drugs Law Intended to Protect the Health of the People Perverted to Protect Adulteration of Foods and Drugs* (Washington, D.C.: Harvey W. Wiley, 1929), pg. 401-402.

[135] Chan PC, Hill GD, Kissling GE, Nyska A. Toxicity and carcinogenicity studies of 4-methylimidazole in F344/N rats and B6C3F1 mice. Arch Toxicol. 2008 Jan;82(1):45-53. Epub 2007 Jul 10. Erratum in: Arch Toxicol. 2008 Jan;82(1):55.

[136] Cavallaro, Matt (2009-06-26). "The Seeds Of A Monsanto Short Play". Forbes.

[137] Dana Hull, 09/01/2012, Monsanto, which is fighting efforts to label genetically engineered food in California, supported labeling such food in Britain, Mercury News,(http://www.mercurynews.com/elections/ci_21452920/monsanto-fighting-efforts-label-genetically-engineered-food-california), Accessed September 12, 2012.

[138] Frost & Sullivan, Introduction to Nutraceuticals, (http://www.frost.com/prod/servlet/cio/236145272), Accessed September 12, 2012.

[139] The Alpha-Tocopherol, Beta Carotene Cancer Prevention Study Group, N Engl J Med 1994 Apr 14;330(15):1029-35.

[140] *Mortality in Randomized Trials of Antioxidant Supplements for Primary and Secondary Prevention*, Vol. 297 No. 8, February 28, 2007 JAMA. 2007;297:842-857.

[141] Tolonen, *Vitamins and Minerals in Health and Nutrition*, pg. 37.

[142] Harold N. Simpson, *Unhealthy Food = Unhealthy People*, pg. 20-21, 30-31.

[143] Anastasia Toufexis, The New Scoop on Vitamins, *Time Magazine*, (6 Apil 1992), pg. 54-59.

[144] Lonn E, Bosch J, Yusuf S, Sheridan P, Pogue J, Arnold JM, Ross C, Arnold A, Sleight P, Probstfield J, Dagenais GR; HOPE and HOPE-TOO Trial Investigators. Effects of long-term vitamin E supplementation on cardiovascular events and cancer: a randomized controlled trial. JAMA. 2005 Mar 16; 293(11): 1338-47.

[145] Marchioli R, Levantesi G, Macchia A, Marfisi RM, Nicolosi GL, Tavazzi L, Tognoni G, Valagussa F; GISSI-Prevenzione Investigators. Vitamin E increases the risk of developing heart failure after myocardial infarction: Results from the GISSI-Prevenzione trial. J Cardiovasc Med (Hagerstown). 2006 May; 7(5): 347-50.

[146] Hendler SS, Rorvik DR, Eds. PDR for Nutritional Supplements. Montvale: Medical Economics Company, Inc.; 2001.

[147] Lim Y, Traber MG. Alpha-Tocopherol Transfer Protein (alpha-TTP): Insights from Alpha-Tocopherol Transfer Protein Knockout Mice. Nutr Res Pract. 2007 winter; 1(4): 247-53. Epub 2007 Dec 31.

[148] Fujita K, Iwasaki M, Ochi H, Fukuda T, Ma C, Miyamoto T, Takitani K, Negishi-Koga T, Sunamura S, Kodama T, Takayanagi H, Tamai H, Kato S, Arai H, Shinomiya K, Itoh H, Okawa A, Takeda S. Vitamin E decreases bone mass by stimulating osteoclast fusion. Nat Med. 2012 Mar 4; 18(4): 589-94.

[149] Berson EL, Rosner B, Sandberg MA, Hayes KC, Nicholson BW, Weigel-DiFranco C, Willett W. A randomized trial of vitamin A and vitamin E supplementation for retinitis pigmentosa. Arch Ophthalmol. 1993 Jun; 111(6): 761-72.

[150] Lehninger, A.L. (2005) *Lehninger principles of biochemistry* (4 th ed.), pg. 768, New York: W.H Freeman.

[151] Sure, Barnett: Influence of Massive Doses of Vitamin B1 on Fertility and Lactation, J. Nutrition 18:187-194 ((Aug.)) 1939.

[152] Los Angeles Times, New Lemon Vitamin Cure for Bleeding, Sunday, March 14, 1937, Editorial Section, Part II, page 1 and page 3.

[153] Vinson J, Bose P, Lemoine L, Hsiao KH. Bioavailability studies. In Nutrient Availability: Chemical and Biological Aspects. Royal Society of Chemistry, Cambridge (UK) 1989:125-127.

[154] Vinson JA, Bose P. Comparative bioavailabililty of humans to ascorbic acid alone or in a citrus extract. IS J Clin Nutr, 1988; 48:601-604.

[155] Vinson JA, Hu S, Jung S. A citrus extract plus ascorbic acid decreases lipids, lipid peroxides, lipoprotein oxidative susceptibility, and atherosclerosis in hypercholesterolemic hamsters. J Agric Food Chem, 1998; 46:1453-1469.

[156] Pesticide News Story: EPA Releases Report Containing Latest Estimates of Pesticide Use in the United States, For Release: February 17, 2011, http://epa.gov/oppfead1/cb/csb_page/updates/2011/sales-usage06-07.html, accessed August 10, 2012.

[157] Bonner MR, Coble J, Blair A, Beane Freeman LE, Hoppin JA, Sandler DP, Alavanja MC. Malathion exposure and the incidence of cancer in the agricultural health study. Am J Epidemiol. 2007 Nov 1;166(9):1023-34. Epub 2007 Aug 23.

[158] Lee WJ, Blair A, Hoppin JA, Lubin JH, Rusiecki JA, Sandler DP, Dosemeci M, Alavanja MC. Cancer incidence among pesticide applicators exposed to chlorpyrifos in the Agricultural Health Study. J Natl Cancer Inst. 2004 Dec 1;96(23):1781-9.

[159] Whitney KD, Seidler FJ, Slotkin TA. Developmental neurotoxicity of chlorpyrifos: cellular mechanisms. Toxicol Appl Pharmacol 134:53-62 (1995).

[160] Eskenazi B, Marks AR, Bradman A, Harley K, Barr DB, et al. 2007 Organophosphate Pesticide Exposure and Neurodevelopment in Young Mexican-American Children. Environ Health Perspect 115(5): doi:10.1289/ehp.9828.

[161] Purdey, Mark, *Journal of Nutritional Medicine*, 1994, 4:43-82.

[162] K Mobed, E B Gold, M B Schenker, Occupational health problems among migrant and seasonal farm workers, West J Med. 1992 September; 157(3): 367–373.

[163] Bretaudeau Deguigne M, Lagarce L, Boels D, Harry P. Metam sodium intoxication: the specific role of degradation products--methyl isothiocyanate and carbon disulphide--as a function of exposure. Clin Toxicol (Phila). 2011 Jun;49(5):416-22

[164] Lifang Hou, Won Jin Lee Jennifer Rusiecki, Jane A. Hoppin, Aaron Blair, Matthew R. Bonner, Jay H. Lubin, Claudine Samanic, Dale P. Sandler, Mustafa

Dosemeci, Michael C. R. Alavanja,Pendimethalin Exposure and Cancer Incidence Among Pesticide Applicators, Epidemiology. 2006 May; 17(3): 302–307.

[165] Crump, Doug; Kate Werry,; Nik Veldhoen,; Aggelen, Van; Caren Helbing,. "Exposure to the herbicide acetochlor alters thyroid hormone-dependent gene expression and metamorphosis in Xenopus laevis." Environmental Health Perspectives. National Institute of Environmental Health Sciences. 2002. *HighBeam Research*. 10 Aug. 2012.

[166] Hayes TB, Collins A, Lee M, Mendoza M, Noriega N, Stuart AA, Vonk A. Hermaphroditic, demasculinized frogs after exposure to the herbicide atrazine at low ecologically relevant doses. Proc Natl Acad Sci U S A. 2002 Apr 16;99(8):5476-80.

[167] Bradberry SM, Proudfoot AT, Vale JA. Glyphosate poisoning. Toxicol Rev. 2004;23(3):159-67.

[168] Lectures by Dr. Royal Lee, Volume I, page 168.

[169] Anabolic steroids and growth hormone, *Am J Sports Med*, June 1993 21 468-474.

[170] Endocrinology: An Integrated Approach; Nussey S, Whitehead S, Oxford: BIOS Scientific Publishers; 2001.

[171] Shaffer EA. Epidemiology and risk factors for gallstone disease: has the paradigm changed in the 21st century? Curr Gastroenterol Rep. 2005 May;7(2):132-40.

[172] New Drugs/Drug News New, P T. 2009 October; 34 (10): 531-534, 541-542.

[173] Reich H. Laparoscopic hysterectomy. Surg Laparosc Endosc. 1992 Mar;2(1):85-8.

[174] Petrovich Z, Ameye F, Baert L, Bichler KH, Boyd SD, Brady LW, Bruskewitz RC, Dixon C, Perrin P, Watson GM. New trends in the treatment of benign prostatic hyperplasia and carcinoma of the prostate. Am J Clin Oncol. 1993 Jun;16(3):187-200.

[175] Gaffney-Stomberg E, Insogna KL, Rodriguez NR, Kerstetter JE. Increasing dietary protein requirements in elderly people for optimal muscle and bone health. J Am Geriatr Soc. 2009 Jun;57(6):1073-9.

[176] Rose WC, Wixom RL, Lockhart HB, Lambert GF. The amino acid requirements of man. XV. The valine requirement; summary and final observations. *J Biol Chem*. 1955; 217:987- 995.

[177] McLagan, Jennifer (2008). *Fat: An Appreciation of a Misunderstood Ingredient*. p. 195.

[178] Morton, Mark (2004). *Cupboard Love: A Dictionary of Culinary Curiosities*. p. 222.

[179] Kabara, J J, THE PHARMACOLOGICAL EFFECTS OF LIPIDS, The American Oil Chemists Society, Champaign, IL, 1978, 1-14; Cohen, L A, et al, J NATL CANCER INST, 1986, 77:43.

[180] Bowden RG, Wilson RL, Deike E, Gentile M. Fish oil supplementation lowers C-reactive protein levels independent of triglyceride reduction in patients with end-stage renal disease. Nutr Clin Pract. 2009 Aug-Sep;24(4):508-12.

[181] Dahlen, G H, et al, J Intern Med, Nov 1998, 244(5):417-24; Khosla, P, and K C Hayes, J Am Coll Nutr, 1996, 15:325-339; Clevidence, B A, et al, Arterioscler Thromb Vasc Biol, 1997, 17:1657-1661.

[182] Lawson, L D and F Kummerow, LIPIDS, 1979, 14:501-503; Garg, M L, LIPIDS, Apr 1989, 24(4):334-9.

[183] Mahadik SP, Evans D, Lal H: Oxidative stress and the role of antioxidant and n-3 essential fatty acid supplementation in schizophrenia. *Prog Neuropsychopharmocol Biol Psychiatry* 2001;25:463-493.

[184] Bourne JM, Dumont O: Essentiality of n-3 fatty acids for brain structure and function. *World Rev Nutr Diet* 1991;66-103-117.

[185] Radenahmad N, Saleh F, Sawangjaroen K, Vongvatcharanon U, Subhadhirasakul P, Rundorn W, Withyachumnarnkul B, Connor JR. Young coconut juice, a potential therapeutic agent that could significantly reduce some pathologies associated with Alzheimer's disease: novel findings. Br J Nutr. 2011 Mar;105(5):738-46. Epub 2010 Nov 30.

[186] Machlin, I J, and A Bendich, FASEB JOURNAL, 1987, 1:441-445.

[187] Van Wagtendonk, W J and R Wulzen, ARCH BIOCHEMISTRY, Academic Press, Inc, New York, NY, 1943, 1:373-377.

[188] S O'Keefe and others. Levels of Trans Geometrical Isomers of Essential Fatty Acids in Some Unhydrogenated US Vegetable Oils. JOURNAL OF FOOD LIPIDS 1994;1:165-176.

[189] MG Enig, Trans Fatty Acids in the Food Supply: A Comprehensive Report Covering 60 Years of Research, 2nd Edition, Enig Associates, Inc., Silver Spring, MD, 1995.

[190] Source: ACE Lifestyle & Weight Management Coach Manual.

[191] The Journal of the American Medical Association, November 7, 1942, page 763.

[192] Bruce GM, Pleus RC, Snyder SA. Toxicological relevance of pharmaceuticals in drinking water. Environ Sci Technol. 2010 Jul 15;44(14):5619-26.

[193] Stackelberg PE, Gibs J, Furlong ET, Meyer MT, Zaugg SD, Lippincott RL. Efficiency of conventional drinking-water-treatment processes in removal of pharmaceuticals and other organic compounds. Sci Total Environ. 2007 May 15;377(2-3):255-72. Epub 2007 Mar 23.

[194] Benotti MJ, Trenholm RA, Vanderford BJ, Holady JC, Stanford BD, Snyder SA. Pharmaceuticals and endocrine disrupting compounds in U.S. drinking water. Environ Sci Technol. 2009 Feb 1;43(3):597-603.

[195] Benachour N, Aris A. Toxic effects of low doses of Bisphenol-A on human placental cells. Toxicol Appl Pharmacol. 2009 Dec 15;241(3):322-8. Epub 2009 Sep 18.

[196] Trasande L, Attina TM, Blustein J. Association between urinary bisphenol A concentration and obesity prevalence in children and adolescents. JAMA. 2012 Sep 19;308(11):1113-21.

[197] Alonso-Magdalena P, Morimoto S, Ripoll C, Fuentes E, Nadal A. The estrogenic effect of bisphenol A disrupts pancreatic beta-cell function in vivo and induces insulin resistance. Environ Health Perspect. 2006 Jan;114(1):106-12.

[198] Cross AJ, Sinha R. Meat-related mutagens/carcinogens in the etiology of colorectal cancer. *Environmental and Molecular Mutagenesis* 2004; 44(1):44–55.

[199] Buts JP, Bernasconi P, Vaerman JP, Dive C. Stimulation of secretory IgA and secretory component of immunoglobulins in small intestine of rats treated with Saccharomyces boulardii. Dig Dis Sci. 1990 Feb;35(2):251–256.

[200] Castex F, Corthier G, Jouvert S, Elmer GW, Lucas F, Bastide M. Prevention of Clostridium difficile-induced experimental pseudomembranous colitis by Saccharomyces boulardii: a scanning electron microscopic and microbiological study. J Gen Microbiol. 1990 Jun;136(6):1085–1089.

[201] Guarner F, Malagelada JR. Gut flora in health and disease. Lancet. 2003 Feb 8;361(9356):512-9.

[202] Sears CL. A dynamic partnership: celebrating our gut flora. Anaerobe. 2005 Oct;11(5):247-51.

[203] 2010 Toxic Release Inventory National Report, US EPA, Office of Toxic Substances.

[204] Pantuck, E.J., Panuck, C. B., Garland, W.A., Mln, B.H., Wattenberg, L.W., Anderson, K.E., Kappas, a., and Conney, A.H. Stimulatory effect of Brussels sprouts and cabbage on human drug metabolism. Clin. Pharmacol. Ther., 25:88-95, 1979.

[205] Mcdanell, R., McLean, A.E.M., Hanley, A.B., Heany, R.K., and fenwick, R.r. Differential induction of mixed function oxidases activity int eh rat liver and intestine by diet containing processed cabbage: correlation with cabbage levels of glucosinolates and glucosinolate hydrolysis products. Food Chem. Toxicol., 25: 363-368, 1987.

[206] Vang. O., Jensen, M.B., and Autrup, H. Induction of cytochrome P-4501A1,1A2,IIB1, and IIE1 by broccoli in rat liver and colon. Chem. Biol. Interact, 78:85-96, 1991.

[207] Wattenberg, L.W. Inhibition of drug-metabolisng enzymes: a path to discovery of multiple cytochrome P450, Annu. Rev. Pharmacol. Toxicol., 43:1-30, 2003.

[208] Ref: Carcinogenesis 2004 25(9):1659-1669.

[209] Kot M, Daniel WA. Effect of cytochrome P450 (CYP) inducers on caffeine metabolism in the rat. Pharmacol Rep. 2007 May Jun;59(3):296-305.

[210] Hutley L, Prins JB. Fat as an endocrine organ: relationship to the metabolic syndrome. Am J Med Sci. 2005 Dec;330(6):280-9.

[211] James P. Powell, Joseph S. LeonardAffiliations, A nutritional program improved lipid profiles and weight in 28 chiropractic patients: a retrospective case series, Journal of Chiropractic Medicine, Volume 7, Issue 3 , Pages 94-100 , September 2008.

[212] U.S. Census Bureau, Statistical Abstract of the United States: 2011, Table 213. Per Capita Consumption of Major Food Commodities: 1980 to 2008, pg. 139.

[213] Mirvish SS. Kinetics of dimethylamine nitrosation in relation to nitrosamine carcinogenesis. J Natl Cancer Inst. 1970 Mar;44(3):633–639.

[214] Y Kurokawa, A Maekawa, M Takahashi, and Y Hayashi, Toxicity and carcinogenicity of potassium bromate--a new renal carcinogen, Environ Health Perspect. 1990 July; 87: 309–335.

[215] www.cdc.gov

[216] http://gaetacommunications.com/site/?p=1092, Accessed August 6, 2012.

[217] Kaygusuz S, Erdemoglu AK, Köksal I. Afebrile convulsion in an adult after recombinant hepatitis B vaccination. Scand J Infect Dis. 2002;34(4):314-5.

[218] Shaw FE Jr, Graham DJ, Guess HA, Milstien JB, Johnson JM, Schatz GC, Hadler SC, Kuritsky JN, Hiner EE, Bregman DJ, et al. Postmarketing surveillance for neurologic adverse events reported after hepatitis B vaccination. Experience of the first three years. Am J Epidemiol. 1988 Feb;127(2):337-52.

[219] Blumberg DA, Lewis K, Mink CM, Christenson PD, Chatfield P, Cherry JD. Severe reactions associated with diphtheria-tetanus-pertussis vaccine: detailed study of children with seizures, hypotonic-hyporesponsive episodes, high fevers, and persistent crying. Pediatrics. 1993 Jun;91(6):1158-65.

[220] Barlow WE, Davis RL, Glasser JW, et al.; Centers for Disease Control and Prevention Vaccine Safety Datalink Working Group. The risk of seizures after receipt of whole-cell pertussis or measles, mumps, and rubella vaccine. *N Engl J Med.* 2001;345(9):656–661.

[221] Dórea JG. Integrating experimental (in vitro and in vivo) neurotoxicity studies of low-dose thimerosal relevant to vaccines. Neurochem Res. 2011 Jun; 36(6): 927-38. Epub 2011 Feb 25.

[222] Park EK, Mak SK, Kültz D, Hammock BD. Evaluation of cytotoxicity attributed to thimerosal on murine and human kidney cells. J Toxicol Environ Health A. 2007 Dec; 70(24): 2092-5.

[223] Vetvicka V, Vetvickova J. Effects of glucan on immunosuppressive actions of mercury. J Med Food. 2009 Oct; 12(5): 1098-104.

[224] National Toxicology Program. Final Report on Carcinogens Background Document for Formaldehyde. Rep Carcinog Backgr Doc. 2010 Jan;(10-5981): i-512.

[225] Fischer MH. THE TOXIC EFFECTS OF FORMALDEHYDE AND FORMALIN. J Exp Med. 1905 Feb 1; 6(4-6): 487-518.

[226] Kumari A, Lim YX, Newell AH, Olson SB, McCullough AK. An XPF-dependent pathway suppresses formaldehyde-induced genome instability. DNA Repair (Amst). 2012 Mar 1; 11(3): 236-46. Epub 2011 Dec 18.

[226] Prival MJ, Peiperl MD, Bell SJ. Determination of combined benzidine in FD & C yellow no. 5 (tartrazine), using a highly sensitive analytical method. Food Chem Toxicol. 1993 Oct; 31(10): 751-8.

[226] Benzidine (Group 1), Evidence for carcinogenicity to humans (*sufficient*) ,http://www.inchem.org/documents/iarc/suppl7/benzidine.html, Accessed July 24, 2012.

[226] Ganguly R, Pierce GN. Trans fat involvement in cardiovascular disease. Mol Nutr Food Res. 2012 Jul; 56(7): 1090-6.

[226] Morris MC, Evans DA, Bienias JL, Tangney CC, Bennett DA, Aggarwal N, Schneider J, Wilson RS. Dietary fats and the risk of incident Alzheimer disease. Arch Neurol. 2003 Feb; 60(2): 194-200.

226 Chavarro JE, Stampfer MJ, Campos H, Kurth T, Willett WC, Ma J. A prospective study of trans-fatty acid levels in blood and risk of prostate cancer. Cancer Epidemiol Biomarkers Prev. 2008 Jan; 17(1): 95-101.

226 Kavanagh K, Jones KL, Sawyer J, Kelley K, Carr JJ, Wagner JD, Rudel LL. Trans fat diet induces abdominal obesity and changes in insulin sensitivity in monkeys. Obesity (Silver Spring). 2007 Jul; 15(7): 1675-84.

226 Chavarro JE, Rich-Edwards JW, Rosner BA, Willett WC. Dietary fatty acid intakes and the risk of ovulatory infertility. Am J Clin Nutr. 2007 Jan; 85(1): 231-7.

226 CS Johnston, CA Gaas. Vinegar: Medicinal Uses and Antiglycemic Effect, MedGenMed, 8(2): 61. May 30 2006.

226 Center for Disease Control andPrevention,
http://www.cdc.gov/nchs/fastats/fertile.htm, Accessed Aug 1, 2012.

226 Center for Disease Control and Prevention,
http://www.cdc.gov/reproductivehealth/Infertility/index.htm, Accessed Aug 1, 2012.

226 Vikis HG, Gelman AE, Franklin A, Stein L, Rymaszewski A, Zhu J, Liu P, Tichelaar JW, Krupnick AS, You M. Neutrophils are required for 3-methylcholanthrene-initiated, butylated hydroxytoluene-promoted lung carcinogenesis. Mol Carcinog. 2011 Oct 17.

226 Shearn CT, Fritz KS, Thompson JA. Protein damage from electrophiles and oxidants in lungs of mice chronically exposed to the tumor promoter butylated hydroxytoluene. Chem Biol Interact. 2011 Jul 15; 192(3): 278-86. Epub 2011 Apr 21.

226 Wiley, Harvey W., M.D., *The History of a Crime Against the Food Law: The Amazing Story of the National Food and Drugs Law Intended to Protect the Health of the People Perverted to Protect Adulteration of Foods and Drugs* (Washington, D.C.: Harvey W. Wiley, 1929), pg. 401-402.

226 Chan PC, Hill GD, Kissling GE, Nyska A. Toxicity and carcinogenicity studies of 4-methylimidazole in F344/N rats and B6C3F1 mice. Arch Toxicol. 2008 Jan; 82(1): 45-53. Epub 2007 Jul 10. Erratum in: Arch Toxicol. 2008 Jan; 82(1): 55.

226 Davis VM, Bailey JE Jr. Chemical reduction of FD&C yellow No. 5 to determine combined benzidine. J Chromatogr. 1993 Apr 9; 635(1): 160-4.

226 International Agency for Research on Cancer (IARC): Benzidine monograph: http://www.inchem.org/documents/iarc/suppl7/benzidine.html, Accessed Aug 3, 2012.

226 Tolonen, *Vitamins and Minerals in Health and Nutrition*, pg. 37.

226 Harold N. Simpson, *Unhealthy Food = Unhealthy People*, pg. 20-21, 30-31.

226 Anastasia Toufexis, The New Scoop on Vitamins, *Time Magazine*, (6 Apil 1992), pg. 54-59.

226 Hendler SS, Rorvik DR, eds. PDR for Nutritional Supplements. Montvale: Medical Economics Company, Inc.; 2001.

[226] Lim Y, Traber MG. Alpha-Tocopherol Transfer Protein (alpha-TTP): Insights from Alpha-Tocopherol Transfer Protein Knockout Mice. Nutr Res Pract. 2007 winter; 1(4): 247-53. Epub 2007 Dec 31.

[226] Fujita K, Iwasaki M, Ochi H, Fukuda T, Ma C, Miyamoto T, Takitani K, Negishi-Koga T, Sunamura S, Kodama T, Takayanagi H, Tamai H, Kato S, Arai H, Shinomiya K, Itoh H, Okawa A, Takeda S. Vitamin E decreases bone mass by stimulating osteoclast fusion. Nat Med. 2012 Mar 4; 18(4): 589-94.

[226] Lonn E, Bosch J, Yusuf S, Sheridan P, Pogue J, Arnold JM, Ross C, Arnold A, Sleight P, Probstfield J, Dagenais GR; HOPE and HOPE-TOO Trial Investigators. Effects of long-term vitamin E supplementation on cardiovascular events and cancer: a randomized controlled trial. JAMA. 2005 Mar 16; 293(11): 1338-47.

[226] Marchioli R, Levantesi G, Macchia A, Marfisi RM, Nicolosi GL, Tavazzi L, Tognoni G, Valagussa F; GISSI-Prevenzione Investigators. Vitamin E increases the risk of developing heart failure after myocardial infarction: Results from the GISSI-Prevenzione trial. J Cardiovasc Med (Hagerstown). 2006 May; 7(5): 347-50.

[226] Berson EL, Rosner B, Sandberg MA, Hayes KC, Nicholson BW, Weigel-DiFranco C, Willett W. A randomized trial of vitamin A and vitamin E supplementation for retinitis pigmentosa. Arch Ophthalmol. 1993 Jun; 111(6): 761-72.

[226] Lehninger, A.L. (2005) *Lehninger principles of biochemistry* (4 th ed.), pg. 768, New York: W.H Freeman.

[226] Sure, Barnett: Influence of Massive Doses of Vitamin B1 on Fertility and Lactation, J. Nutrition 18:187-194 ((Aug.)) 1939.

[226] Los Angeles Times, New Lemon Vitamin Cure for Bleeding, Sunday, March 14, 1937, Editorial Section, Part II, page 1 and page 3.

[226] Vinson J, Bose P, Lemoine L, Hsiao KH. Bioavailability studies. In Nutrient Availability: Chemical and Biological Aspects. Royal Society of Chemistry, Cambridge (UK) 1989:125-127.

[226] Vinson JA, Bose P. Comparative bioavailability of humans to ascorbic acid alone or in a citrus extracts. Am J Clin Nutr, 1988; 48:601-406.

[226] Vinson JA, Hu S, Jung S. A citrus extract plus ascorbic aciddecreases lipids, lipid peroxides, lipoprotein oxidative susceptibility, and atherosclerosis in hypercholesterolemic hamsters. J Agric Food Chem, 1998; 46:1453-1469.

[226] www.cdc.gov.

[226] http://gaetacommunications.com/site/?p=1092, Accessed August 6, 2012.

[226] Dórea JG. Integrating experimental (in vitro and in vivo) neurotoxicity studies of low-dose thimerosal relevant to vaccines. Neurochem Res. 2011 Jun; 36(6): 927-38. Epub 2011 Feb 25.

[226] Park EK, Mak SK, Kültz D, Hammock BD. Evaluation of cytotoxicity attributed to thimerosal on murine and human kidney cells. J Toxicol Environ Health A. 2007 Dec; 70(24): 2092-5.

[226] Vetvicka V, Vetvickova J. Effects of glucan on immunosuppressive actions of mercury. J Med Food. 2009 Oct; 12(5): 1098-104.

226 National Toxicology Program. Final Report on Carcinogens Background Document for Formaldehyde. Rep Carcinog Backgr Doc. 2010 Jan;(10-5981): i-512.

226 Fischer MH. THE TOXIC EFFECTS OF FORMALDEHYDE AND FORMALIN. J Exp Med. 1905 Feb 1; 6(4-6): 487-518.

226 Kumari A, Lim YX, Newell AH, Olson SB, McCullough AK. An XPF-dependent pathway suppresses formaldehyde-induced genome instability. DNA Repair (Amst). 2012 Mar 1; 11(3): 236-46. Epub 2011 Dec 18.

227 http://www.dddmag.com/news/2009/11/bms-splits-mead-johnson-nutrition, Accessed April 29, 2013.

228 Aniansson G, Alm B, Andersson B, and et al. "A prospective cohort studies on breast-feeding and otitis media in Swedish infants". Pediatr Infect Dis J. 1994; 13:183-188.

229 Kovar MG, Serdula MK, Marks JS, et al. "Review of the epidemiologic evidence for an association between infant feeding and infant health." Pediatrics. 1984:74:S615-S638.

230 Stuebe A. The risks of not breastfeeding for mothers and infants. Rev Obstet Gynecol. 2009 Fall; 2(4): 222-31.

231 Mayer, EJ, Hamman RF, Gay EC, et al. "Reduced risk of IDDM among breast-fed children". Diabetes, 1988; 37:1625-1632.

232 Burch-Johnson, K., et al., "Relation between breastfeeding and incidence of insulin-dependent diabetes mellitus". Lancet 2:1083-86 (1984).

233 Davis MK, Savitz DA, Graubard BI. "Infant feeding and childhood cancer." Lancet. 1988; 2:365-368.

234 Shu X-O, Clemens H, Zheng W, et al. "Infant breastfeeding and the risk of childhood lymphoma and leukaemia". Int J Epidemiol. 1995; 24:27-32.

235 Ford RPK, Taylor BJ, Mitchell EA, et al. "Breastfeeding and the risk of sudden infant death syndrome. Int J. Epidemiol. 1993; 22:885-890.

236 Mitchell EA, Taylor BJ, Ford RPK, et al. "Four modifiable and other major risk factors for cot death: the New Zealand Study". J Paediatr Child Health. 1992; 28:S3-S8.

237 Lucas A., "Breast Milk and Subsequent Intelligence Quotient in Children Born Preterm". Lancet 1992; 339:261-62.

238 Lucas A, Brooke OG, Morley R, et al. "Early diet of preterm infants and development of allergic are atopic disease: randomized prospective study". Br Med J. 1990:300:837-840.

239 Halken S, Host A, Hansen LG, et al. "Effect of an allergy prevention programme on incidence of atopic symptoms in infancy". Ann Allergy. 1992; 47:545-553.

240 Freudenheim, J. et al. 1994 "Exposure to breast milk in infancy and the risk of breast cancer". Epidemiology 5:324-331.

INDEX

ABOUT THE AUTHOR

Gerald Roliz is an aspiring hunter-gatherer. He enjoys eating healthy foods, drinking pristine spring water and breathing fresh air. All of which can be found in the outdoors. In overcoming nature-deficit disorder, Gerald Roliz is a unique member of a global hunter-gatherer tribe, who are rewilding the intuitive essence of humanity. He enjoys freedom from the technological advances of society with long hikes, meditation with nature and foraging for wild foods. He is fascinated by the opportunities for primal exploration which transform modern day citizens into paleo-humanitarians. May you find your path to wellness. He looks forward to meeting you along the journey of life.

Made in the USA
San Bernardino, CA
25 October 2013